Treatment of Communication Disorders in Culturally and Linguistically Diverse Populations

CONTRIBUTORS

Boris E. Bogatz, Ph.D.
Interim Dean
School of Education and Human Services
Gallaudet College
Washington, DC 20002

Margaret Forbes, M.S.
University of Pittsburgh
Department of Communication
Pittsburgh, PA 15260

Toshi Hisama, Ph.D.
Associate Professor
Department of Special Education
Southern Illinois University at Carbondale
Carbondale, IL 62901

Audrey Holland, Ph.D.
University of Pittsburgh
Department of Communication
Pittsburgh, PA 15260

John L. Manni, Ed.D.
Director, Psychological Services
Irving Schwartz Institute for Children and Youth
Philadelphia, PA 19131

Harry N. Seymour, Ph.D.
University of Massachusetts
Department of Communication Disorders
Amherst, MA 01003

Orlando L. Taylor, Ph.D.
Howard University
School of Communications
Department of Communication Arts and Sciences
Washington, DC 20059

Fay Boyd Vaughn-Cooke, Ph.D.
University of the District of Columbia and Center for Applied Linguistics
Department of Communication Sciences
Washington, DC 20001

Reesa G. Wurtz, Ed.D.
Assistant Professor
Department of School Psychology
Temple University
Philadelphia, PA 19122

Treatment of Communication Disorders in Culturally and Linguistically Diverse Populations

Edited by

Orlando L. Taylor, Ph.D.
Howard University

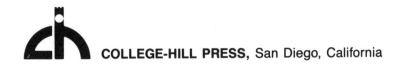

COLLEGE-HILL PRESS, San Diego, California

College-Hill Press, Inc.
4284 41st Street
San Diego, California 92105

Library of Congress Cataloging in Publication Data
Main entry under title:

Treatment of communication disorders in culturally and linguistically diverse
    populations.
    Companion vol. to Nature of communication disorders in culturally and
linguistically diverse populations.
    Includes indexes.
    1. Communicative disorders — Treatment.   2. Language disorders —
Treatment.   3. Language and culture.   4. Linguistic minorities.   I. Taylor,
Orlando L., 1936-   . II. Nature of communication disorders in culturally and
linguistically diverse populations.   III. Title.
RC423.T74   1986   616.85'5   85-224-31
ISBN 0-88744-221-8
Printed in United States of America

To LeRoy and Carrie Taylor, my Father and Mother

CONTENTS

PREFACE

Since the early 1970s, there as been considerable discussion on how to identify and treat pathological communicative behaviors in the various cultural and linguistic groups that reside in the United States of America. In addition to the field of communication disorders, much of this discussion has centered on research in such disciplines as sociolinguistics, bilingual education, and cognitive psychology on such diverse topics as (1) culturally valid — and legal — assessment of linguistic, communicative, and cognitive function, (2) culturally appropriate techniques for delivering clinical services to individuals with speech and language disorders, and (3) culturally sensitive and effective pedagogies for teaching standard English as a second language.

Each of these issues is represented in this volume. Although numerous articles and monographs have been published on the various clinical topics outlined, to date no book has been published that presents a critical, comprehensive review of them and provides specific proposals for future directions for the discipline of communication directions with respect to cultural and linguistic diversity.

At the outset, the book was intended to be a single volume on the nature of normal communicative behavior in culturally and linguistically diverse populations and approaches for valid assessment and management of communication disorders within these populations. Once the project was undertaken in early 1984, it became obvious that the body of literature was too great to be addressed adequately in a single volume. Consequently, two books were written — this book and a companion volume, *Nature of Communication Disorders in Culturally and Linguistically Diverse Populations.*

This book is divided into three parts: Part I, consisting of one chapter, focuses on background issues pertaining to cultural and linguistic diversity. Part II, consisting of three chapters, focuses on the assessment of speech and language disorders in culturally and linguistically diverse populations. Part III, consisting of three chapters, focuses on management and educational issues, using the nonstandard English speaker as a case study.

In Chapter 1, the editor discusses the historical factors associated with the issue of cultural and linguistic diversity within the field of communication disorders and presents a conceptual framework for viewing the issue of diversity. In this chapter, the author describes the positions taken in the late 1960s and early 1970s by scholars and practitioners, during which time the various cultural issues were being named within the discipline. These descriptions are continued through 1985, when the American Speech-Language-Hearing Association sponsored a National Colloquium on Underserved Populations. The chapter concludes with the presentation of a model for viewing normal and pathological communication from a framework that takes into account the social, cognitive, and communicative norms of the culture from which a person comes.

In Chapter 2, Fay Vaughn-Cooke discusses the urgent professional need for developing appropriate assessment procedures for evaluating speech and language function in non-standard English speakers. Vaughn-Cooke evaluates the eight most frequently presented alternatives to traditional assessment procedures for persons whose cultural or linguistic communities are outside the white, middle class American mainstream. The chapter ends with a presentation of six criteria to be used for constructing new alternatives to inappropriate diagnostic tests.

In Chapter 3, Audrey Holland and Margaret Forbes propose several assessment alternatives to standardized testing for culturally and linguistically diverse populations. Among the procedures they discuss are spontaneous language samples, language probes, and various structured elicitation tasks. Holland and Forbes place particular attention on functional or pragmatic profiles for determining a person's communicative competence within a specific language system.

Chapter 4, by Boris Bogatz and several of his colleagues, presents a comprehensive discussion of the issues involved in nondiscriminatory cognitive assessment of nonwhite children that result in poor identification of individuals in need of special education services and, more particularly, in poor evaluation of cognitive deficiencies associated with communication disorders. Bogatz and colleagues explore legal considerations correlated with basic available assessment alternatives. They conclude with an elucidation of an extensive model for implementing a nondiscriminatory process for all types of evaluations.

In Chapters 5 and 6, companion chapters by Harry Seymour, the issue of management of communication disorders in non-standard English speakers is addressed. In these two comprehensive chapters, Seymour proposes six clinical principles to be employed in approaching the question of clinical intervention with persons who come from non-standard English speech communities. He argues that every learning plan for language disordered children must be (1) multidimensional, (2) interactional, (3) generative, (4) bidialectal, (5) child-centered, and (6) diagnostic. In Chapter 6, Seymour shows how these six principles articulate with intervention goals, the determination of causation and symptoms, the testing of hypotheses about a child's language through a language probing process (LPP), and available methods for altering disordered language behavior among non-standard English speakers.

Chapter 7, written by the editor, addresses educational issues associated with teaching standard English as a second dialect. Taylor touches on the historical and legal issues associated with this topic, together with the models which have been advanced to teach standard English to non-standard English speaking people. After stating why these methods have generally failed, Taylor describes his field-tested alternative to these traditional methods. Using a communicative versus a linguistic model, he outlines his cultural and communicative approach, code named ACCPT, which is built around six major tenets: (1) an oral focus, (2) a communicative orientation, (3) an interactional focus of structure, function, and thought, (4) a linkage to products, (5) a linkage across the curriculum, and (6) a linkage to a developmental teaching model. Sample lessons and evaluation strategies are also included.

The book ends with a postscript on where the discipline of communication disorders needs to move to more effectively serve the needs of the complete cultural mosaic of the United States of America — indeed, of the world.

Some may take issue with this book on the grounds that not all cultural and ethnic groups in the United States are sufficiently covered. In a sense, this criticism is valid, especially with respect to the obvious omission of substantial materials on Asian Americans, the nation's fastest growing immigrant population. At the same time, it should be noted that the literature is relatively small for many of these other populations. Moreover, the book is written as a case study in what we know about a select group of the most populous nonwhite populations in the United States. It is hoped that this book will stimulate more publications from others on other groups, as well as on the peoples covered herein.

Finally, the reader is encouraged to read the companion volume, *Nature of Communication Disorders in Culturally and Linguistically Diverse Populations*. This book discusses specific assessment, management, and educational issues pertaining to culturally and linguistically diverse persons. Major chapters cover (1) anthropological and sociolinguistic considerations in the study of communications, (2) language variation in the United States, (3) language acquisition in culturally diverse populations, and (4) the prevalence and nature of communication disorders in Black Americans, Hispanics, Native Americans, and several indigenous peoples of North America.

ACKNOWLEDGMENTS

As editor, I wish to express sincere thanks to my numerous friends and colleagues at Howard University and throughout the country for their support and encouragement during the preparation of this book. Special appreciation is extended to the members of my loyal and dedicated staff for their inspiration and assistance in preparing the final manuscript, and to all the members of my immediate family for their unequivocal love through the years. Finally, but certainly not least in importance, I wish to acknowledge the stimulation and motivation I have received from many students during the past 20 years at Indiana University, Federal City College (University of the District of Columbia), Stanford University, and particularly Howard University. My scholarship is a reflection of my continuing intellectual commitment to you.

PART I
BACKGROUND

Chapter 1

Historical Perspectives and Conceptual Framework

Orlando L. Taylor

Prior to 1968, little interest was shown within the professions of speech pathology and audiology in addressing the unique clinical needs of individuals with communication disorders from culturally and linguistically diverse populations. With respect to speech-language function, professionals tended to have a poor perception of the distinction between a legitimate linguistic *difference* and a speech-language *disorder*. Moreover, virtually all norms within all subspecialties of communication were based on what we might call a middle class, Euro-American model.

In this introductory chapter, we examine some of the historical events, legal decisions, legislative initiatives, and research findings that have resulted in significant changes in how professionals in communication disorders have come to view the nature of these disorders in culturally and linguistically diverse populations. The chapter concludes with the presentation of a conceptual framework for examining this topic.

THE WINDS OF CHANGE: THE 1968 ASHA CONVENTION

In 1968, a very important event occurred at the Annual Convention of the American Speech and Hearing Association (ASHA) in Denver, Colorado. The ASHA President, John V. Irwin, in a bold change from tradition, decided to forego the annual Presidential Address to permit a debate between Orlando L. Taylor of Indiana University and John Michel of the University of Kansas on "The Role of a Professional Association in a Conflict Society." Irwin's courageous act grew out of severe national discord over the Vietnam war and civil unrest by Blacks in numerous urban centers.

Michel took the position that professional associations should not be involved in social issues.

> It is unwise to jeopardize the purely professional nature of ASHA and the harmony among our Members by introducing current issues outside the realm of speech and hearing . . . . It is both healthy and admirable that individual Members are sensitive to social issues and have the courage to organize opinion against unsatisfactory aspects of our society.

> (Michel, 1969, p. 220)

Taylor took an opposite position. He argued, in part, that

> professional organizations should articulate a point of view on the important social and political issues of the day, making it possible for the corporate body to influence decisions . . . . I urge the American Speech and Hearing Association to provide aggressive leadership for moral, ethical and judicial behavior in areas of social significance.
> (Taylor, 1969, p. 217)

The Michel-Taylor debate stimulated great discussion and exchange within the professions of speech pathology and audiology. Out of this dialogue came enormous changes, which serve as a backdrop for addressing the topic of communication disorders within culturally and linguistically diverse populations.

THE EMERGENCE OF THE ASHA BLACK CAUCUS

The most immediate and, at the time, the most important outgrowth of the Michel-Taylor debate at the 1968 ASHA Convention was the formation of a Black Caucus. This caucus of the majority of the then minuscule Black membership (probably less than 100 persons) addressed several concerns in a special report (Taylor, Stroud, Hurst, Moore, and Williams, 1969) to the ASHA membership.

One of the three major objectives of the ASHA Black Caucus was to urge the Association to

> encourage appropriate research and curriculum revisions in the area of urban language behavior, most of which is black language, to the extent that more intelligent clinical and educational services can be made available to black children.
> (Taylor et al., 1969, p. 222)

Speaking to the language objectives more specifically, the ASHA Black Caucus established two related goals:

1. To urge ASHA to require coursework in sociolinguistics (and Black history) for clinical certification.
2. To urge ASHA to organize a committee to generate new ideas on training and research in sociolinguistics, especially as related to Black language.

Addressing the first goal, the ASHA Black Caucus wrote

Unfortunately, far too many speech pathologists view legitimate language differences among Afro-Americans from a pathology model. The result is that a number of black children are receiving speech and language therapy, particularly in urban areas, when they, in fact, have no pathology. Negative psychological effects on the black child are obvious. In order to develop a more intelligent approach to recognizing legitimate linguistic differences and satisfactory methods for second language instruction as a skill, clinicians need training in sociolinguistics (interaction between language and culture) and the historical and cultural roots of black children. All too often clinicians fail to understand the black child's language, as well as the child himself.

(p. 224)

On the second goal, the ASHA Black Caucus asserted

Even if ASHA required institutions to offer a course in sociolinguistics, there is a dearth of knowledge about language, its patterns of acquisition, and viable means for utilizing it for teaching standard English as a skill. Likewise, there is a dearth of qualified teachers in this area. ASHA might assume some leadership in terms of training personnel (clinicians and teachers) for work in this area and stimulating the basic and applied research needed. It is noteworthy that a number of other professionals have already begun serious work in urban language, e.g., linguists, sociologists, and teachers of English. Unless the profession of communication disorders begins to put forth a major thrust in this area, it will lose a great opportunity to catapult itself into an arena of great educational and cultural interest.

(p. 224)

ASHA AND THE PROFESSION RESPOND

Largely in response to the aforementioned Michel-Taylor debate and the advocacy by the ASHA Black Caucus, a number of important actions have been taken within the profession of communication disorders since 1969 to address the needs of clinically and linguistically diverse populations. Among the most important of these actions are the following:

1. ASHA opened an Office of Urban and Ethnic Affairs in 1969 (this office was changed to the Office of Minority Concerns in 1979).
2. ASHA established Committees on Communication Behaviors and Problems in Urban Populations in 1969 (now the Committee on Cultural and Linguistic Differences and Disorders of Communication) and on the Status of Racial Minorities in 1973.
3. Several symposia, colloquia, and continuing education activities have been presented throughout the United States on normal and clinical issues pertaining to culturally and linguistically diverse populations. ASHA'S 1985 National Colloquium on Underserved Populations is a good example of this type of activity.
4. ASHA has taken official positions on social dialects, and on the clinical management of communicatively handicapped minority language populations. (Position papers on each are presented in the Appendix.) The social dialects position recognizes the legitimacy of all dialects of a language, as well as the validity of a linguistic standard. A specific role is outlined for speech pathologists in teaching standard English to *normal* speakers, and the qualifications needed by the professional who engages in this activity are noted. The communicatively handicapped minority language statement outlines national clinical needs in this area, a continuum of language proficiency, professional competencies for bilingual speech pathologists, and strategies for procuring competent personnel to provide clinical services to bilingual persons.
5. Several universities have inaugurated special training projects to address the specific clinical needs of culturally or linguistically diverse populations — for example, University of Arizona (Native Americans); San Diego State University, Temple University, and University of the District of Columbia (Bilingual Populations); and Howard University (Black American and Third World Populations).
6. Presentations in professional meetings and publications in professional journals have increased dramatically since 1969 on a myriad of topics pertaining to cultural and linguistic diversity. For example, Cole (1985) reports that at the 1984 ASHA Convention, over 50 sessions focused on minority issues. This percentage represented a 100 percent increase over 1982 and a 5,000 percent increase over 1969, when there was only one session on this topic. Regrettably, some of this research on minority issues still contains negative views and invalid assumptions on cultural and linguistic divergence.

LEGAL AND LEGISLATIVE DEVELOPMENTS

Concurrent with the activities within the American Speech-Language-Hearing Association, a number of legal and legislative actions occurred during the 1970s and 1980s that have influenced issues on cultural and linguistic diversity in the field of communication disorders. Some of these actions will be discussed in this section.

The fourteenth amendment to the United States Constitution guarantees, in part, that all citizens are entitled to receive equal protection under the law. This entitlement was defined operationally in Title VI of the Civil Rights Act of 1964. Title VI states

> No person in the United States shall, on the ground of race, color, or national origin, be excluded from participation in, be denied benefits of, or be subjected to discrimination under any program or activity receiving federal financial assistance.

Several significant court decisions were made during the 1970s that cited the fourteenth amendment and Title VI as bases for ruling on behalf of plaintiffs in cases that had enormous impact on the field of communication disorders. These decisions led, in turn, to several important legislative actions (see Table 1–1).

Table 1-1. Major Legislative Actions

Civil Rights Act of 1964, United States Congress, Title VI. 1964.

Bilingual Education Act of 1968, United States Congress.

Public Law 94–142, The Education of All Handicapped Children Act. (November 29, 1975).

Public Law 95–561, The Bilingual Education Act of 1976.

U.S. Code of Federal Regulations, Number 34, Part 300. 532 (a), 1973.

The most important decision was *Lau v. Nichols* (1974). In this landmark case, the Supreme Court ruled unanimously in favor of the plaintiffs from San Francisco's Chinatown community, who claimed that the absence of programs designed to meet their specific linguistic needs violated their civil rights. The plaintiffs argued further, and the Court agreed, that equality of education goes beyond the provision of the same buildings and books to all students to include intangible factors such as language. Because they could not understand the English language used in the classroom, the Chinese plaintiffs argued, they were deprived of even a minimally adequate, and hardly equal, education. In addition, they asserted that the equal rights provision of the United States Constitution prohibited withholding from them the means of comprehending the language of instruction from any citizen (Center for Applied Linguistics, 1977).

The importance of *Lau v. Nichols* to the field of communication disorders, and to bilingual education, was that it established unequivocally that the handling of language differences in public facilities, or those receiving Federal funds, fell within the purview of constitutional guarantees pertaining to equal rights and to Civil Rights legislation. *Lau v. Nichols* led to the passage of the Bilingual Education Act of 1976, and to several additional lawsuits pertaining to the rights of persons who speak a language other than English (e.g., *Serna v. Portales Municipal Schools,* 1974, in New Mexico; *Aspira v. Board of Education of the City of New York,* 1974).

Citing *Lau v. Nichols* and Section 1703(f) of Title 20 of the United States Code, a United States District Judge in Michigan ruled in 1979 on behalf of nine Black children in Ann Arbor who claimed that the local school board had denied them their equal rights by failing to take their native Black English into account in the educational process (*Martin Luther King Junior Elementary School Children, et al., v. Ann Arbor School District Board,* 1978). Section 1703(f) of Title 20 states

> No State shall deny equal educational opportunity to an individual on account of his or her race, color, sex, or national origin by . . .
>
> (f) the failure of an educational agency to take appropriate action to overcome language barriers that impede equal participation by its students in its instructional programs.

Since the Ann Arbor School Board did not appeal this ruling, the decision on behalf of the nine children and their parents did not have the effect of federal law. However, it did establish the legitimacy of the claim that dialect variation, like language differences, could not be used to discriminate against children in the implementation of educational programs.

Several other court decisions and legislative actions have spoken even more directly to issues affecting clinical practices in communication disorders. Most have involved issues of assessment procedures used to identify and place children into speech-language therapy and into special and compensatory education classes. It is well documented that children from linguistic and cultural minorities tend to be placed into special education and related services at higher rates than their representation in local school populations. In some cases, however, there is an underrepresentation in these classes and services (Jones and Cartwright, 1981). In either event, inappropriate testing and other assessment procedures are thought to be the cause of the problem.

Three court decisions in state and federal courts have supported the notion that discriminatory testing procedures cannot be used to place children in special education classes and related services. These cases are *Dianna v. Board of Education* (1973) (California); *Larry P. v. Wilson Riles* (1977) (California); and *Mattie T. v. Holladay* (1977) (Mississippi).

The Education of All Handicapped Children Act of 1975, Public Law 94–142, and its revision, PL 98–199, provide the most explicit language to date that outlaws the use of discriminatory testing to place children in special education classes and in such related services as speech, language, and hearing therapy. Section 34:300.532 (a) of the U.S. Code of Federal Regulations (1983) pertaining to the provisions of PL 94–142 and 98–199 states

> State and local educational agencies shall insure, at a minimum, that:
> (a) Tests and other evaluation materials:
> (1) Are provided and administered in the child's native language or other mode of communication, unless it is clearly not feasible to do so.

These various legal decisions and legislative initiatives in the past two decades have established legitimacy to the claim that a child's native language system has to be considered in the development and implementation of special education programs and in the provision of clinical services to communicatively impaired persons. Moreover, they have provided a basis for advocates of culturally and linguistically diverse populations to couch their claims in legal terms, in addition to academic and intellectual terms.

RESEARCH DEVELOPMENTS

As stated earlier, research issues pertaining to communication disorders in culturally and linguistically diverse populations have increased dramatically since the 1960s. This research, which has come from many disciplines, has provided the underpinnings for the present state of the art with respect to our understanding of the treatment of communication disorders in culturally and linguistically diverse populations.

In general, the studies of particular value to the study of this topic have focused on such topics as the following:

1. culturally valid assessment procedures of cognitive, linguistic, and communicative behaviors;
2. the nature and prevalence of communication disorders in a vari-

ety of cultural and linguistic groups in the United States and around the world; and

3. cultural and linguistic issues in the delivery of clinical services.

In subsequent chapters of this book, much of this research will be discussed critically. For now, however, we may state seven conclusions that might be drawn from this research literature to serve as general principles undergirding studies of the treatment of communication disorders in culturally and lingustically diverse populations. These conclusions are as follows:

1. Valid, legal, and ethical communication assessment must take into account the cognitive, linguistic, communicative, and social rules emanating from the culture from which the person being assessed comes (Terrell and Terrell, 1983).
2. Societies differ with respect to what they consider normal and pathological communicative behavior. Despite these differences, it appears that virtually all types of communication disorders, particularly those with organic causes, exist within all cultures in the world (Taylor, 1980).
3. Cultures around the world tend to place different values on the presence of communication disorders and the priorities they place on their remediation (Taylor and Samara, 1985).
4. The prevalence and incidence of various communication disorders differ in various cultures, depending on such variables as genetic factors, social and environmental conditions, quality of health care, societal definitions of what is considered pathological, epidemiology of various diseases and syndromes, and diet.
5. The nature of speech-language disorders within a given language or dialect group can be defined validly only from the vantage point of linguistic and communicative norms of that language or dialect (Mercer, 1983; Wolfram, 1983).
6. The treatment of communication disorders within a given cultural group should take into account the cultural and communicative norms of the client, his or her preferred learning styles, the linguistic and communicative characteristics of the targeted language or dialect, the values placed on communication disorders by the client's cultural group, and the culturally defined roles of the client.
7. A nonstandard dialect should not be construed as a speech or language disorder. A speaker of nonstandard language can be taught the standard variety of a language, particularly if he or she wishes to learn that variety. Instruction in a second dialect is an *educational*, not a *clinical*, activity, which must follow a set of cul-

turally based principles and pedagogical strategies to be successful (Taylor, 1985).

A CONCEPTUAL FRAMEWORK

Professional, legal, and research developments in communication disorders and related disorders, particularly those since the 1960s, permit us to devise a culturally based framework for studying the nature — and the treatment — of communication disorders in culturally and linguistically diverse populations. The framework devised by this author is schematized in Figure 1–1.

As shown in Figure 1–1, the basic premise of this author's conceptual framework is that the study of normal and pathological communication must be couched in cultural terms. To do otherwise is to run the risk of making claims and judgments about the communicative behaviors of a given group of speakers from an inappropriate or, even worse, an ethnocentric set of assumptions and norms. The omnipresence of culture is demonstrated in Figure 1–1 by virtue of the placement of all four processes and outcomes germane to the study of the nature and treatment of communication pathology within the boundaries of culture.

The four processes and outcomes that operate within the constraints of culture are (1) developmental issues, (2) precursors of communication pathology, (3) assessment and diagnosis, and (4) treatment. The first two processes speak to the nature of communication disorders within a given cultural group. Processes three and four speak to clinical issues of diagnosis and management.

These processes are listed hierarchically in terms of their importance in addressing issues in communication disorders. The outcomes, although presented sequentially, are necessarily artificially ordered inasmuch as many components of each process are likely to develop simultaneously with one another.

Process 1 — Developmental Issues

Developmental processes provide the foundation for understanding the nature and treatment of communication disorders within any cultural or linguistic group. Two levels of development are presented: (1) development within the indigenous culture, and, following the likely exposure to outside cultures, (2) optional development of external cultural, cognitive, language and communicative behaviors. In the model, solid lines denote expected phenomena, whereas dashed lines denote optional phenomena.

The four outcomes of the developmental process *within* the indigenous culture include (1) adult-child interaction within the culture,

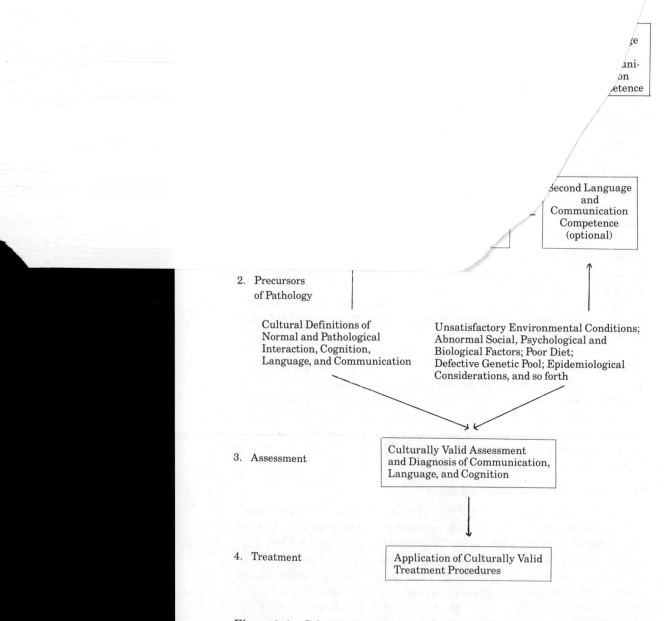

ge
ani-
on
etence

Second Language
and
Communication
Competence
(optional)

2. Precursors
   of Pathology

Cultural Definitions of
Normal and Pathological
Interaction, Cognition,
Language, and Communication

Unsatisfactory Environmental Conditions;
Abnormal Social, Psychological and
Biological Factors; Poor Diet;
Defective Genetic Pool; Epidemiological
Considerations, and so forth

3. Assessment

Culturally Valid Assessment
and Diagnosis of Communication,
Language, and Cognition

4. Treatment

Application of Culturally Valid
Treatment Procedures

Figure 1-1. Schematic view of a culturally based conceptual framework for studying and treating communication disorders in culturally and linguistically diverse populations.

(2) cognitive acquisition within the framework of a specific culture, (3) the acquisition of indigenous language and communication systems, and (4) the development of adult language and communicative competence.

The foundation for all indigenous culture development is thought to be the adult-child interactions that occur within the sociocultural context of a specified group. These interactions provide a model for the developing child for, among other things, acceptable cognitive, linguistic, and communicative behaviors. Through this early socialization, the child is believed, at least by some, to develop a set of culturally and socially based concepts and thoughts (Vygotsky, 1962). This underlying conceptual development gives rise, in turn, to the acquisition of verbal and nonverbal symbols (language) and rules for using them (communication), within the rules of the indigenous culture. Over time, through practice, increased socialization, and biological maturation, the child is expected to acquire adult language and communication competence within the norms established by the indigenous culture.

Although possible, it is highly unlikely, at least in the economically developed world, for the developing child to be so culture bound that he or she is never exposed to external cultures. If nothing else, modern mass communication systems and compulsory education guarantee some type of external cultural exposure. This optional external cultural interaction is shown through a set of dashed lines emanating from each of the four basic processes of indigenous cultural development. These connections with the box labeled *external culture interactions* show that the optional (though likely) exposures to other cultures may occur at any stage of the developmental process from infancy through adulthood.

The final stage of developmental outcomes involves *optional* development, which might occur in a person (child or adult) as a result of external cultural interactions. These outcomes, which are schematized in the lower tier of the developmental outcomes in Figure 1–1, may be thought of as *second* cognitive, language, and communication acquisition. The occurrence and degree of acquisition of external or second systems are dependent on a number of social, political, and psychological factors (e.g., age of exposure, degree of exposure, relative political and social power of the indigenous and external cultures, motivation for acquiring the external culture, and method of acquiring the second culture). In any case, this second tier of outcomes recognizes the possibility that an individual may acquire, at varying levels of competence, the cognitive, linguistic, and communicative systems of another culture, as a replacement for or addition to his indigenous culture, or as a hybrid of the two. Since language is intimately linked with thought, Figure 1–1 suggests that any type of cognitive acquisition within the external culture will necessarily lead to some level of acquisition of the language and communication of the external culture. As shown by the dashed lines, however, it is not necessarily the case that adult competence will result in either area.

Process 2 — Precursors of Pathology

Normal cognitive, linguistic, and communication development may not occur in a given individual even under the best of cultural conditions. There are two major precursors to the emergence of communication pathology, or at least to what individuals consider to be communicatively pathological within a given culture. The first might be called "culturally defined pathological behaviors." The second set of precursors includes the whole array of abnormal or unsatisfactory biological, social, psychological, nutritional and genetic factors that are known to contribute to the development of communication pathology.

In viewing these precursors of communication pathology, however, the reader is reminded that cultural factors assume an enormously important role in the definition of what is considered pathological. Culture also determines the definition of the quality and *normalcy* of an environment, diet, social condition, psychological state, or even a biological condition.

The role of cultural definitions of communication pathology cannot be overemphasized. Scattered observations from around the world reveal that societies have different perceptions of what they consider pathological communication and, equally important, what to do about it when it does exist. Taylor and Samara (1985) claim that some societies believe that little or nothing should be done about communication disorders, except to keep them hidden from the public. In some cases, these disorders are thought to be acts of God(s) or demons. In Arabic speaking countries, for example, this concept exists and is referred to as "kikmat Rabana."

With this cultural notion in mind, it seems reasonable to argue that based on what is known about the social and cultural dimensions of the form, content, and use of language by people around the world, it is obvious that a communication disorder in any society can only be defined from the vantage point of the speech community of which a given speaker is a member. Therefore, a strong claim can be made that such "standard" definitions of communication disorders, such as the one advanced by Van Riper (1978), should be revised to something like the following:

> Communicative behavior by an individual can only be considered defective if it deviates sufficiently from the norms, expectations, and definitions of his or her indigenous culture (or language group); that is, if it is
>
> (a) considered to be defective by the indigenous culture or language group;
>
> (b) operates outside the minimal norms of acceptability of that culture or language group;
>
> (c) interferes with communication *within* the indigenous culture or language group;
>
> (d) calls attention to itself within the indigenous culture or language group, or
>
> (e) causes the user to be "maladjusted" as defined by the indigenous culture.

With respect to the standard list of causative factors associated with communication pathology, the point must be reiterated that although the causative factors listed in Figure 1–1 probably exist all over the world, cultural factors influence the values and perceptions that interact with them. For example, a poor diet in one culture may be considered to be a good diet in another culture. Likewise, one culture's view of a satisfactory social environment may be another culture's perception of a completely unacceptable social environment.

Epidemiological considerations as a precursor of communication disorders deserve special attention in this discussion. All too often, the communication disorders specialist determines the relative importance of various diseases and syndromes as etiological factors from within the framework of their prevalence of distribution within his or her given culture. In truth, however, the relative importance of various diseases and syndromes as etiological factors in communication disorders should vary from culture to culture. Thus, within the United States, it is probably appropriate to place considerable attention on such medical conditions as stroke, closed head injuries, and cancer as examples of major causes of communication disorders. In other parts of the world, however, other medical conditions might be considered more important. For example, in much of the Third World, great emphasis might be placed on schistosomiasis* as a dis-

---

*Petersdorf and colleagues (1983) describe schistosomiasis as a water-carried parasitic disorder that affects the gastrointestinal system, the liver, and the vascular system and causes central nervous system damage. Over 200,000,000 persons are thought to be afflicted with this disease in more than 71 countries, virtually all in the developing world, although the disorder is probably being brought to Europe and North America by immigrant populations. There are no reports in the literature on the effects of schistosomiasis on speech, language, or hearing function, despite its capacity to cause vascular obstructions and CNS damage.

ease that contributes to the onset of communication disorders. In Africa, and in countries throughout the world where African descendants now reside, sickle cell disease might be considered to be a major cause of hearing loss and, therefore, the recipient of considerable professional attention.

Process 3 — Assessment

The third conceptual notion of the model in Figure 1–1 addresses the need for culturally and linguistically valid testing and other assessment procedures for determining communication pathology within individuals from a specified culture or language group. As stated earlier in this chapter, culturally valid procedures are required by federal law to conform with what many would consider to be ethical practice in the field of communication disorders.

Culturally valid assessment, by definition, includes the use of test instruments and other formal and informal procedures for collecting linguistic and communicative data from an individual, for determining the level of development, or for determining the presence of abnormality. These assessments must be conducted from the vantage point of the indigenous or preferred system of communication of the person being assessed. If group comparisons are to be made, they must be made in the context of standards or norms derived from comparable individuals from the same cultural or linguistic group as the client.

The entire Spring, 1983, edition of *Topics in Language Disorders* provides an excellent discussion of nonbiased assessments of communicative behaviors. In that volume, Taylor and Payne (1983) observe, quite accurately, that when a researcher wishes to construct culturally valid assessment instruments and procedures, controls must be carefully chosen to prevent the emergence of several sources of potential bias: linguistic, format, situational, examiner, values, and directions.

Finally, Taylor (1985) has argued that culturally valid assessment procedures should

1. Recognize that clients may perform differentially under differing clinical conditions because of their cultural and language backgrounds.
2. Recognize that different modes, channels, and functions of communication events in which individuals are expected to participate in a clinical setting may result in differing levels of linguistic or communicative performance.

3. Use ethnographic techniques for evaluating communicative be-
    havior and establishing cultural norms for determining the pres-
    ence or absence of communication disorders.

Process 4 — Treatment

Finally, the conceptual framework schematized in Figure 1–1
suggests that when it has been validly determined that an individual from a given culture has a communication disorder, culturally
and linguistically valid therapy may ensue. Given the cultural orientation of the model, it goes almost without saying that treatment
must be in the context of the values, attitudes, and wishes of the indigenous culture relative to communication disorders and what to do
about them. Treatment should also take into account the preferred
learning style of the client and the rules of social and communicative interaction as defined by the client's indigenous cultural or linguistic group.

Taylor (1985) claims that all clinical encounters are cultural
events and, as such, the clinician should develop an ethnological approach to all clinical practice. In addition to the principles mentioned in Process 3, he claims that clinicians should

1. View each clinical encounter as a socially situated communica-
    tive event that is subject to the cultural rules governing such
    events by both the clinician and the client.
2. Recognize possible sources of conflicts in cultural assumptions
    and communicative norms in clients prior to clinical encounters,
    and take steps to prevent them from occurring during service
    delivery.
3. Recognize that learning and culture are on-going processes that
    should result in a constant reassessment and revision of ideas
    and greater sensitivity to cultural diversity.

Finally, culturally valid clinical treatment uses culturally appropriate materials, activities, and subject matters of high interest,
which are packaged within intervention strategies compatible with
the preferred learning styles of the client's culture.

SUMMARY

In this chapter, we presented an overview of some of the major
historical, legal, legislative, and research issues that undergird the
study of the nature of communication disorders in culturally and lin-

guistically diverse populations. A culturally based conceptual framework was also presented for viewing developmental, etiological, assessment, and treatment issues for these same populations.

This conceptual framework forms the basis for much of this volume and should be referred to as the reader addresses various issues pertaining to the nature of communication disorders within culturally and linguistically diverse populations.

REFERENCES

Aspira of New York, Inc., v. Board of Education of the City of New York, 72 Civ. 4002 (S.D.N.Y. August 29, 1974) (unreported consent decree).

Center for Applied Linguistics (1977). *Bilingual education: Current perspectives (law).* Washington, DC: Author.

Cole, L. (1985). ASHA Interviews. *ASHA, 27,* 23–25.

Dianna v. State Board of Education, C.A. 70 RFT (N.D. Cal., Feb. 3, 1970).

Jones, R. R., and Cartwright, L. R. (1981). *National survey: Foreign speakers in speech and hearing clinics.* Paper presented at the Annual Convention of the American Speech and Hearing Association, Los Angeles.

Larry P. v. Wilson Riles, Civil Action No. 0-71-2270, 343 F. Supp. 1306 (N.D. Cal., 1972).

Lau v. Nichols, 411 U.S. 563 (1974).

Mattie T. v. Holladay, 522 F. Supp. 72 (N.D. Miss., 1977).

Martin Luther King Junior Elementary School Children, et al., v. Ann Arbor School District Board, Civil Action No. 7-71861, 451 F. Supp. 1324 (1978), 463 F. Supp. 1027 (1978) and 473 F. Supp. 1371 (1979) Detroit, Michigan (1979).

Mercer, J. R. (1983). Issues in the diagnosis of language disorders in students whose primary language is not English. *Topics in Language Disorders, 3,* 43–56.

Michel, J. F. (1969). The role of ASHA in social, political, and moral activities. *ASHA, 11,* 219–220.

Petersdorf, R. G., Adams, R. D., Braunwald, E., Isselbacher, K. J., Martin, J. B., and Wilson, J. D. (1983). *Harrison's principles of internal medicine.* New York: McGraw-Hill.

Serna v. Portales Municipal Schools, 351 F. Supp. 1279 (N.D. Mex. 1972) aff'd, 499 F. 2d 1147, 1154 (10th Cir. 1974).

Taylor, O. (1969). Social and political involvement of the American Speech and Hearing Association. *ASHA, 11,* 216–218.

Taylor, O., Stroud, R., Hurst, G., Moore, E., and Williams, R. (1969). Philosophies and goals of the ASHA Black Caucus. *ASHA, 11,* 221–225.

Taylor, O. (1980). *Communication disorders in Blacks.* Proceedings of International Conference on Communication. New York: The Rockefeller Foundation.

Taylor, O., and Payne, K. (1983). Culturally valid testing: A proactive approach. *Topics in Language Disorders, 3,* 8–20.

Taylor, O., and Samara, R., (1985). *Communication disorders in underserved populations: Developing nations.* Paper presented at the National Colloquium on Underserved Populations, American Speech and Hearing Association, Washington, DC.

Taylor, O. (in press). Clinical practice as a social occasion: An ethnographic model. *ASHA Reports.*

Terrell, S. L., and Terrell, F. T. (1983). Distinguishing linguistic differences from disorders: The past, present, and future of non-biased assessment. *Topics in Language Disorders, 3,* 1–7.

Van Riper, C. (1978). *Speech Corrections.* Englewood Cliffs, NJ: Prentice-Hall.

Vygotsky, L. V. (1962). *Thought and language.* Ed. and Tr. by E. Hanfmann and G. Vakar. Cambridge, MA: MIT Press.

Wolfram, W. (1983). Test interpretation and sociolinguistic differences. *Topics in Language Disorders, 3,* 8–20.

PART II
THE ASSESSMENT OF SPEECH AND LANGUAGE DISORDERS IN CULTURALLY AND LINGUISTICALLY DIVERSE POPULATIONS

Chapter 2

The Challenge of Assessing the Language of Nonmainstream Speakers

Fay Boyd Vaughn-Cooke

One of the most critical and urgent problems facing professionals in the field of speech and language pathology today is the absence of adequate assessment tools needed to provide valid and reliable evaluations of the language varieties spoken by nonmainstream speakers. This problem has existed for more than half a century—ever since speech and language pathology has been recognized as a field of study. Its significance, however, was not acknowledged until the late 1960s and early 1970s, when it was illuminated by a small but determined group of language researchers (Adler, 1971; Baratz, 1969a, 1969b; Wolfram, Williams, and Taylor, 1972), who argued that the varieties of English spoken by nonmainstream speaker exhibit linguistic features that differ from the standard variety and that such features should not be viewed as deviant when assessing the language of nonmainstream speakers.

The implications of this position were far-reaching. Revolutionizing the process of assessing the language of nonmainstream speakers was required. A major change would have involved abandoning the use of all assessment procedures that viewed standard English features as the only normal and acceptable linguistic structures. Professionals would have had to discontinue using almost every language assessment device available at the time in the fields of speech and language pathology. Of course this was not done. Inappropriate tests continued to be and still are administered to nonmainstream speakers, but the reasons for abandoning them are compelling and overwhelming. Thus, an intense search has been sparked for alternatives to tests that are capable of assessing the language only of Standard English speakers. The goal of this chapter is to (1) examine and evaluate these alternatives, and (2) present some basic guidelines for developing additional alternatives.

ALTERNATIVES TO INAPPROPRIATE SPEECH AND LANGUAGE TESTS FOR NONMAINSTREAM SPEAKERS

The following alternatives have been proposed by various scholars and practitioners to assess speech and language functions in nonmainstream speakers:

1. Continue to use existing standardized assessment tools.
2. Standardize existing tests on nonmainstream English speakers.
3. Include a small percentage of minorities in the standardization sample when developing a test.
4. Modify or revise existing tests in ways that will make them appropriate for nonmainstream speakers.
5. Use a language sample when assessing the language of nonmainstream speakers.
6. Use criterion-referenced measures when assessing the language of nonmainstream speakers.
7. Refrain from using all standardized tests that have not been corrected for test bias when assessing the language of nonmainstream speakers.
8. Develop new tests that can provide more appropriate assessments of the language of nonmainstream speakers.

These alternatives will be discussed and evaluated in turn.

Continue Using Existing Inappropriate Standardized Assessment Tools

Although this alternative has not been formally recommended in the recent literature on assessment, practitioners are forced to adopt it regularly in clinical and educational settings around the country. Such tools as the Illinois Test of Psycholinguistic Abilities (ITPA) (Kirk, McCarthy, and Kirk, 1968) and the Peabody Picture Vocabulary Test (PPVT) (Dunn and Dunn, 1981) are still used when assessing the language of nonmainstream English speakers.

The PPVT was employed as part of a learning disabilities assessment for one of the plaintiff children in the 1979 Ann Arbor case, a nationally publicized court case relating to use of Black English (*Martin Luther King Junior Elementary School Children et al. v. Ann Arbor School District Board, 1979*). Excerpts from the results of the assessment reported in the second amended complaint by the counsel for the plaintiffs included the following:

> The Peabody Picture Vocabulary Test measures the student's language receptive skills. . . . From the results obtained from this evaluation, her [the plaintiff's] language receptive skills are at the lower limits of the average range of intelligence. Her mental age of 5.4 years in . . . contrast to 3.8 years of age when she was evaluated . . .
>
> (Kaimowitz and Lewis, 1979, p. 10)

Regarding the ITPA, this test was used frequently in the 1960s and 1970s in research studies, and results consistently revealed that Black, nonstandard English speaking children scored lower than their standard English speaking counterparts (Arnold and Read, 1976; Larson and Olson, 1963; Lively-Weiss and Koller, 1973; McConnell, Horton, and Smith, 1969; Rychman, 1967; Smith and May, 1967; Stephenson and Gay, 1972. Nonmainstream speakers can pay a great price when invalid assessment tools are used; Wolfram's item analysis (1980, 1983) of the Grammatic Closure Subtest of the ITPA dramatically illustrates this point. Consider the following table, which provides a comparison of "correct" responses (as required by the scoring procedure) and the possible responses from nonmainstream English speakers.

Table 2–1 shows that *only* standard English responses are scored as correct on the Grammatic Closure Subtest of the ITPA. Consequently, as many as 24 of the 33 responses from a nonmainstream English speaker could be scored as incorrect. Obviously, the assessor would be forced to conclude that the testee's language was not normal for his or her particular age level. The failure to provide equal credit for nonstandard responses is a serious linguistic flaw underlying the Grammatic Closure Subtest and most standardized language tests. This problem renders all such tools invalid, and any alternative that requires their use must be rejected.

Standardize Existing Tests on Nonmainstream Speakers

This alternative has been adopted by a number of researchers (Evard and McGrady, 1974; Evard and Sabers, 1974; Evard and Sabers, 1979), and it is reflected in several unpublished works in progress. Evard and his associates have standardized the Templin-Darley Tests of Articulation and the Auditory Association and the Grammatic Closure Subtest of the ITPA on nonmainstream speakers in

Table 2-1. ITPA Grammatical Closure Subtest with Comparison of Correct Responses and Vernacular Black English Alternate Forms

Stimulus with Correct Item (Italicized) According to ITPA Test Manual	Possible Response from a Black Nonmainstream English Speaker
1. Here is a dog. Here are two *dogs/doggies*.	dog
2. This cat is under the chair. Where is the cat? She is *on* (any preposition — other than "under" — indicating location).	
3. Each child has a ball. This is hers, and this is *his*.	
4. This dog likes to bark. Here he is *barking*.	
5. Here is a dress. Here are two *dresses*.	dress
6. The boy is opening the gate. Here the gate has been *opened*.	open
7. There is milk in this glass. It is a *glass of/with/for/o'/lots of milk*.	
8. This bicycle belongs to John. Whose bicycle is it? It is *John's*.	John
9. This boy is writing something. This is what he *wrote/has written/did write*.	writed
10. This is the man's home, and this is where he works. Here he is going to work, and here he is going *home/back home/to his home*.	
11. Here it is night, and here it is morning. He goes to work first thing in the morning, and he goes home first thing *at night*.	
12. This man is painting. He is a *painter/fence painter*.	
13. The boy is going to eat all the cookies. Now all the cookies have been *eaten*.	ate
14. He wanted another cookie, but there weren't *any/any more*.	none/no more
15. This horse is not big. This horse is big. This horse is even *bigger*.	more bigger
16. And this horse is the very *biggest*.	most biggest
17. Here is a man. Here are two *men/gentlemen*.	mans/mens
18. This man is planting a tree. Here the tree has been *planted*.	
19. This is soap, and these are *soap/bars of soap/more soap*.	soaps
20. This child has lots of blocks. This child has even *more*.	
21. And this child has the *most*.	mostest
22. Here is a foot. Here are two *feet*.	foots/feets
23. Here is a sheep. Here are lots of *sheep*.	sheeps
24. This cookie is not very good. This cookie is good. This cookie is even *better*.	*gooder*
25. And this cookie is the very *best*.	
26. This man is hanging the picture. Here the picture has been *hung*.	hanged
27. The thief is stealing the jewels. These are the jewels that he *stole*.	stoled/stealed
28. Here is a woman. Here are two *women*.	womans/womens

Table 2-1 (continued).

29. The boy had two bananas. He gave one away and he kept one for *himself.*	hisself
30. Here is a leaf. Here are two *leaves.*	leafs
31. Here is a child. Here are three *children.*	childrens
32. Here is a mouse. Here are two *mice.*	mouses
33. These children all fell down. He hurt himself, and she hurt herself. They all hurt *themselves.*	theirselves/ theyselves theirself/theyself

From Wolfram, W. (1983). Test interpretation and sociolinguistic differences. *Topics in Language Disorders, 3,* 21–34. Reprinted with permission.

Arizona. The raw scores were analyzed according to (1) the norms for standard English speakers, (2) combined norms for four ethnic-racial groups (Anglo-Americans, Black Americans, Mexican-Americans, and Papago Indians) in Arizona, and (3) specific norms for each ethnic-racial group. The results were predictable; the analysis demonstrated successive decreases in the number of children identified as speech and language impaired as the norms became increasingly more specific for each group.

At first glance, standardization of existing tests appears to be a reasonable alternative to use of inappropriate tests, but close scrutiny of the situation reveals that solving the technical problem of standardizing a test can create some irresolvable substantive problems. The first is low norms. The norms, for example, on the Grammatic Closure Subtest would be much lower for Black nonmainstream speakers than for their standard English speaking contemporaries (Wolfram, 1983). Lower norms are a serious shortcoming of this alternative. DeAvila and Havassy (1974) explain why:

> Ethnic norms are potentially dangerous from the social perspective because they provide a basis for invidious comparisons between racial groups. The tendency is to assume that lower scores are indicative of lower potential, thereby contributing to the self-fulfilling prophecy of lower expectations for minority children and reinforcing the genetic-inferiority argument advanced by Arthur Jensen and others.
>
> (p. 72)

The question that needs to be addressed is "Why does the standardization alternative result in lower norms?" The answer to this question exposes the second substantive problem — that is, most standardized language tests, particularly the Grammatic Closure Subtest, are constructed to reveal what a child knows only about standard English. It follows, then, that if speakers are learning standard English in their speech community, they will know a lot (considering age and normal development) and their norms will reflect this, but if speakers are learning nonmainstream varieties, their norms will reflect this fact also. The point is that if a test has been constructed to assess only one dialect of English, standardizing it on children who speak a different dialect will not make it valid or appropriate. For this reason the standardization alternative is not always a viable one.

Include a Small Percentage of Minorities in the Standardization Sample when Developing a Test

This alternative is closely related to the foregoing and it exhibits similar problems. The standardization sample of the ITPA highlights these problems. The ITPA normative sample included 962 children from five Midwestern cities ranging in population from 27,000 to 126,000. The socioeconomic status of the children's families was reported as approximating the distribution in the communities selected and in the nation as a whole. Only about 4 percent of the children were Black. According to Weiner and Hoock (1973), this was lower than the percentage in the communities selected and obviously lower than the percentage of Blacks in the nation. What was accomplished, in terms of validity, by including a small percentage of Blacks in this sample? Nothing, according to Weiner and Hoock (1973). They note

> ... there is a question concerning the decision to include a small Black group in the [ITPA] sample. This group is representative of Black children neither in the communities involved nor in the nation as a whole. Just whom these children do represent is unclear. It might have been better not to include them at all, for they simply reduce the extent to which the sample represents the "average" white population. If they were to be included, a carefully drawn independent sample of "average" Black children would need to be collected and compared with the "average" white group. Only then could the test be used with confidence on Black subjects, using the same norms for all "average" children.
>
> (p. 621)

Weiner and Hoock's (1973) comments point to the inadequacies of this third alternative, which was indeed adopted in the revised version of the PPVT. Blacks represented only 10 percent of the 4,200 nationwide standardization sample. A subsample of this type that is not controlled for social class — a critical variable that affects language — contributes nothing to solving the problem of invalid assessment of minority children's language. Speech-language pathologists should be aware of this fact.

Another, more recent test that adopted the alternative of including a small percentage of minorities in the standardization sample is the Basic Language Concepts Test (BLCT) (Englemann, Ross, and Bingham, 1982). The more than 2,500 children in the BLCT sample included 144 Headstart children and 183 minority group children. These latter two groups constituted the "poverty sample" of Englemann and colleagues. When these investigators compared the poverty population to the general population (the bulk of the sample), they found that

> Children in the poverty groups (both white and minority) had a significantly higher mean number of errors across all parts of the test. Our figures show that these children in the disadvantaged group scored 21–23 months behind the others in their mastery of language skills as measured on the BLCT. The performance pattern suggests that these poverty children are developing normally but are significantly delayed in their mastery of skills.
>
> (Bingham and Ross, 1984, p. 1)

The above quote is very telling. It reveals that Bingham and Ross (1984) have completely missed the point regarding what is required to provide valid language assessments for nonmainstream speakers. No test, irrespective of the percentage of minorities included in the sample, is valid if its results indicate that nonmainstream speaker are 21 to 23 months *behind* their mainstream peers. It is clear that the principles underlying the BLCT evolved from the deficit theory; thus, this test should be avoided by assessment specialists who are committed to using tests that provide substantive, as opposed to superficial and unacceptable, alternatives to inappropriate assessment tools.

Modify or Revise Existing Tests in Ways that Will Make Them Appropriate for Nonmainstream English Speakers

This alternative was adopted by Nelson (1976), and Hemingway, Montague, and Bradley (1981). Nelson modified the scoring procedure for Lee's Developmental Sentence Scoring Technique (DSS) (1974). This technique provides a method for analyzing eight categories of standard English grammatical form. These include indefinite pronouns (e.g., *this, that, some, nothing, anything*), personal pronouns (e.g., *mine, himself, herself, themselves*), main verbs (e.g., copula forms like *is, are, was*), secondary verbs (e.g., *to see, to play, running, broken*), negative forms (e.g., *not, are not*), conjunctions (e.g., *and, but, be-*

cause), interrogative reversal question types (e.g., *Does he still have it?*), and wh-questions (e.g., *Where is the boy?*). Data for the DSS analysis consist of a set (50 or more) of complete sentences (i.e., constructions exhibiting a subject and a verb, which are extracted from spontaneous speech samples). Following Lee's procedure (1974), only standard English responses are scored as correct. Nelson modified the scoring system in an attempt to make the technique appropriate for Black nonmainstream English speakers. The following description indicates how this was done.

> In the development of the BES [Black English Score] chart, two scores were assigned for each BE [Black English] feature. One was a conservative score ... For example, uninflected verbs such as "have/has" would score "1" instead of "2" on the DSS chart, but at least they would score. A second, lenient, score was assigned and bracketed, which gave the full DSS credit which would have been earned if the structure had been generated according to SE [standard English] rules. That is ... [following the lenient scoring] the uninflected verb "have" with third person singular subjects, e.g., "He have a new coat," would score "2." (Nelson, 1976, pp. 6 to 7).

It is important to note that the conservative scores (the lower scores) were used when Nelson (1976) conducted the statistical analysis for her study. According to Nelson, the lower score was used to "avoid over-crediting the Black child for features which are similar to early developing SE [standard English] features" (p. 7).

Any revision which does not provide *equal* credit for comparable nonmainstream and standard English forms is inadequate. Irrespective of the revisers' intentions, a conservative scoring system can be interpreted negatively (i.e., that nonmainstream forms are not "good" enough to receive full credit, as standard English forms would). The concept that *all* dialects are equal must be fully reflected in every aspect of revised versions of traditional tools before they can be viewed as viable alternatives for assessing the speech or language of nonmainstream speakers.

It should be noted that Nelson has developed a revised version of the BESS (Nelson, 1983); however, specific details regarding its scoring system were not presented in her description of the new version.

Like Nelson, Hemingway, Montague, and Bradley (1981) adopted the revision alternative and provided a modification of the Carrow Elicited Language Inventory (CELI) (Carrow, 1974) for assessing the language of 5 and 6 year old Black nonstandard English speakers. The children were asked to repeat 20 sentences from the original CELI. The goal was to use revised requirements that would not penalize speakers if they produced characteristic Black English responses.

This goal is well motivated but, to achieve it, a thorough knowledge of the structure of Black English is required. Unfortunately, such knowledge is not reflected in the Black English responses that are considered acceptable by Hemingway and colleagues. Consider their proposed, acceptable response to item 17 on the modified CELI:

17.   If it rains we won't go to the beach.
      (original test sentence)

      Is it rain we won't go to the beach.
      (Acceptable Black English sentence,
      according to Hemingway et al.)

Although research has shown that it is acceptable for a Black English speaker to say *rain* instead of *rains*, there is no evidence to support the contention that such speakers say *is* instead of *if*. The second construction is ungrammatical and unacceptable in Black English. At least eight of the 20 Black English sentences proposed by Hemingway and colleagues were unacceptable. It is critical that test modifiers obtain a thorough knowledge of nonmainstream dialects *before* initiating revisions. If this is not done the revised versions of traditional tests will be inadequate and thus unacceptable alternatives for nonmainstream speakers.

Use a Language Sample when Assessing the Language of Nonmainstream Speakers

This nonstandardized alternative to assessing the language of minority children has been recommended by a number of researchers, including Leonard and Weiss (1983); Reveron (1983); Seymour and Miller-Jones (1981); Shuy and Staton (1982); Stockman and Vaughn-Cooke (1981), and Vaughn-Cooke (1979,1980). The language sample technique involves collecting a spontaneous speech sample (at least 50 utterances) from a child and conducting an analysis of his or her utterances. The content, structure, and function of the utterances provide some of the crucial evidence needed to determine whether a child's language is developing normally. Language sample analyses play an important role in the assessment of all children's language, but when used as an alternative for assessing the language of nonmainstream children at least two problems arise.

The first is that language sample analyses cannot provide some of the critical information required to make a diagnosis regarding the normalcy of a child's language. For this reason, they must be used in conjunction with appropriate standardized tests, which are generally not available for nonmainstream speakers. Leonard, Perozzi, Prutting, and Berkeley (1978) noted, quite correctly, that such tests serve at least one valuable purpose: "They separate the impaired language user from the normal language user" (p. 373). The first step, then, in the assessment process is to administer a norm-referenced test that can separate, validly and reliably, normal language from disordered language. Language sample analyses cannot accomplish this goal. Diagnosticians should be aware of this limitation.

The second reason why language sample analyses are, at present, not acceptable alternatives to the assessment problem is that the results from such analyses must be interpreted within a developmental framework. Such a framework would reveal the sequence of normal language behaviors for specific age levels. This important sequence evolves from in-depth studies of the development of language in the normal child. Extensive work has been done that has contributed to a well-documented sequence for young, white, middle class children, but the limited number of language acquisition studies on nonmainstream English speaking children precludes the establishment of a valid developmental sequence. At present most of the language behaviors revealed by language sample analyses of nonmainstream speakers must be interpreted according to the sequences established for middle class white children. This is obviously unacceptable; language sample analyses cannot be viewed as viable alternatives until *after* language development research on nonmainstream children has been expanded.

Use Criterion-Referenced Measures when Assessing the Language of Nonmainstream Speakers

This second nonstandardized approach is being recommended as an alternative to inappropriate standardized tests by a growing set of professionals (Bailey and Harbin, 1980; Bergquist, 1982; Drew, 1973; Duffy, Salvia, Tucker, and Ysseldyke, 1981; Seymour and Miller-Jones, 1981; Taylor and Payne, 1983; Ysseldyke and Regan, 1980). Within the context of language assessment, criterion-referenced testing involves specifying the specific linguistic behaviors to be tested and establishing criteria for acceptable responses. A child's responses, however, are not generated for the purpose of comparison with other children's performance. This is the goal of standardized or norm-referenced testing.

Criterion-referenced testing can play an important role in assessment and language intervention, but at present the use of this approach presents one of the problems associated with language sample analyses. There is no valid developmental sequence that can be used to specify which linguistic behaviors should be selected as goals for a particular child. It was noted earlier that the use of a sequence evolved from the study of ethnic and racial groups that are not the same as the child's is unacceptable. Drew's observation is relevant here; he noted

> Criterion-referenced evaluation is not . . . totally free from bias vulnerability. From the standpoint of minority children's evaluation one must also be concerned with criterion-referenced evaluation, particularly in terms of the external referent criterion. Indeed the criterion referent relates most specifically to an instructional goal. This is desirable since, perhaps for the first time, the link between evaluation and instruction is obvious. One must, however, ask the question "What is the criterion and who specifies the criterion to be attained?" As soon as this question is addressed the possibility of subgroup advantage or disadvantage becomes evident.
>
> (p. 327)

The conclusion drawn about criterion-referenced testing is the same as that for language sample analyses: It cannot be viewed as a viable alternative to the assessment problem until *after* language development research on nonmainstream speakers has been expanded.

Refrain from Using All Standardized Tests that Have Not Been Corrected for Test Bias when Assessing the Language of Nonmainstream Speakers

A moratorium on standardized testing has been called by a number of professional organizations and researchers who have debated the assessment issue. The task force on language and communication skills, which met at the National Invitational Symposium on the King Decision (also called the Ann Arbor Decision) at Wayne State University, recommended that the following tests should not be used in the assessment process for Black English speakers:

> Peabody Picture Vocabulary Test, Houston Test of Language Development, Utah Test of Language Development, Grammatic Closure Subtest of the ITPA, Developmental Sentence Scoring Technique, Templin Darley Tests of Articulation, Wepman Test of Auditory Discrimination.

Specifically, the task force concluded

> We . . . call for a moratorium on the use of all of the above tests until new tests are developed and/or revisions made to render such tests ap-

propriate for Black English speakers. Revision should involve expanding the set of acceptable linguistic responses to include Black English structures. Additionally revisions should involve the establishment of test norms for the target population of Black English speakers.

(Daniel and Scott, 1981, p. 310)

Other calls for a moratorium on the use of standardized tests have come from the NAACP and the Association of Black Psychologists. Duffy and colleagues reported that the NAACP, at its 1974 meeting, called for an end to standardized testing if such tests have not been corrected for cultural bias. According to Duffy and colleagues, a similar position was taken by the Council for Exceptional Children Delegate Assembly at its 1978 international convention. The Association of Black Psychologists also maintained that standardized tests should not be used to test minority children. The following position was put forth in Williams (1970):

> The Association of Black Psychologists fully supports those parents who have chosen to defend their rights by refusing to allow their children and themselves to be subjected to achievement, intelligence, aptitude and performance tests which have been and are being used to: A. Label Black people as uneducable. B. Place Black children in "special" classes and schools. . . .

(p. 5)

The moratorium alternative clearly is not the solution to the assessment problem, and its proponents appear to be aware of this. Their goal is to dramatize the issue and highlight the urgent nature of the situation.

Develop New Tests that Can Provide a More Appropriate Assessment of the Language of Nonmainstream Speakers

A number of researchers viewed this proposal as the only solution to the assessment problem (Drumwright, Van Natta, Camp, Frankenburg, and Drexler, 1973; Politzer, Hoover, and Brown, 1974; Williams, 1972). They invested the time and resources to develop completely new tests. Williams (1972) developed the language-based Black Intelligence Test of Cultural Homogeneity (BITCH), Drumwright and colleagues (1973) constructed the Denver Articulation Screening Exam (DASE), and Politzer and colleagues (1974) developed a Test of Proficiency in Black Standard and Nonstandard Speech. Each test will be described briefly and evaluated in turn.

According to Williams (1972), the BITCH is a culture-specific test. The author pointed out that the test is "not intended to be a culture-fair or a culture-common test" (p. 6). The purpose of the test is to assess adolescents' and adults' knowledge of primarily slang terms used by Blacks in various parts of the country. The test constructor reported that the terms were selected from the *Dictionary of Afro-American Slang,* the Word in the *APGA Journal,* friends, and his personal experiences gained from living and working in the Black community. Below is a sample item from the test:

> Item 3.
> Blood
>> (a)   a vampire
>> (b)   A dependent individual
>> (c)   An injured person
>> (d)   A brother of color

The test taker is instructed to select the correct answer (d) from among the four possibilities. Williams' analysis of test scores obtained by 200 Black and white high school students revealed that the former group's scores were significantly higher than the latter's.

The BITCH makes an important point — that is, tests that have been developed to assess specific knowledge exhibited by one cultural group are not appropriate for other cultural groups. The ability to make this point is the only positive feature of the BITCH. Since the test focuses on slang, a very variable and superficial aspect of a speaker's linguistic system, it provides no means for assessing knowledge of the fundamental components of language (semantic, pragmatics, phonology, syntax). It is important to note that this was not the goal of the test; thus, language diagnosticians should not view this tool as an alternative to traditional standardized tests.

Drumwright et al. (1973) maintain that the DASE is an articulation-screening test for economically disadvantaged children. The test, which contains 34 phonemes, was administered to over 1,500 white, Black, and Mexican-American children who ranged in age form 2 years 6 months to 6 years. Each subgroup constituted about one third of the total population tested; thus, the minority standardization sample is one of the largest reported for a language test.

Although the DASE solves some problems for the two groups of nonmainstream speakers, of standardization in particular, it creates others. The most critical is the failure to provide an assessment of a number of phonemes that are generated by nonmainstream phonological rules. The authors' criteria for selecting the 34 phonemes which were included in the test excluded final /ə/, as in *bath* and final /l/, as in *ball.* Final /ə/ can be replaced by /f/ in the nonmainstream variety spoken by many Black children and /l/ can be vocalized (the vowel in the word is then lengthened), which is generally perceived as a deletion. The authors excluded both /ə/ and /l/ from the DASE original list of sounds. The following quote explains why.

Because our aim was an articulation-screening test which would mini-mize incorrect referrals of economically disadvantaged children, we decided to eliminate from the final analysis any sounds which: (1) were not correctly produced by at least 70% of children in all cultural groups by age six. . . .

(p. 8)

The above mentioned criterion indicates that the authors view only the standard English productions of /ə/ and /l/ as correct. Non-mainstream replacements, /f/ and /∅/, are considered incorrect. The test constructors noted that "Only 36% of Black children produced the sound [final /ə/] correctly by age six" (p. 8). Regarding /l/, it was reported: "Only 50% of Black children pronounced the sound cor-rectly" (p. 8). The elimination of structures that can be replaced by nonmainstream variants is unacceptable because this can result in the failure to refer a child for language intervention when it is needed. Once a structure is eliminated, deviant productions cannot be documented. For example, if a nonmainstream English speaker said /f/ for final /ə/, his response would be normal; however, if he said /s/ for final /ə/, his response would be deviant. An articulation test must be able to capture this critical distinction. As noted above, test constructors must obtain a detailed description of the language vari-ety to be evaluated before they initiate the development of new tests.

The DASE problems discussed above can be solved if it is revised to account for dialect variation. After revision it could serve as an appropriate screening-articulation tool for nonmainstream English speakers.

The Test of Proficiency in Black Standard and Nonstandard Speech was designed to measure the ability of children to speak both nonstandard and standard English. The test employs a repetition model; subjects are required to repeat 30 sentences, 15 standard and 15 nonstandard. The test was administered to 35 kindergarten chil-dren; however, the results were not reported for individual subjects. The proficiency test, although developed for Black children, was not constructed to distinguish between normal and deviant linguistic behavior. For this reason it should not be considered as an alterna-tive to traditional standardized tests.

The above discussion of seven alternative approaches for assess-ing the language of nonmainstream speakers reveals a rather dis-mal picture. Unfortunately, the picture is accurate. It is not an over-statement to say that a crisis exists in the area of assessment for nonmainstream speakers. Researchers, clinicians, and test developers must intensify their efforts to overcome this crisis and meet the needs of assessment specialists. These professionals do not need more evaluations of the assessment problem, nor do they need more "interim" solutions. They need valid, reliable assessment tools. To meet this need more tools will have to be constructed. Before the construction process is initiated test developers should carefully consider the criteria, which have been stated implicitly and explicitly throughout the assessment literature, for developing valid assessment tools. Some of these criteria will be discussed in the next section.

SOME CRITERIA FOR CONSTRUCTING NEW ALTERNATIVES TO INAPPROPRIATE TESTS

Some of the alternatives discussed in the preceding section indicate that the professional in communication disorders who wishes to respond to the challenge of providing appropriate assessment tools for nonmainstream speakers must fully understand what is required to meet this challenge. The requirements are complex because the challenge is complex. It was noted earlier that simple strategies, such as including a small percentage of minorities in a standardization sample of a test, are inadequate and accomplish little, except to mislead hopeful practitioners searching for appropriate tools. The goal of this section of the chapter is to present come guidelines that might be helpful to professionals who are in a position to accept the challenge of developing new tests that can provide alternatives to inappropriate ones.

The following criteria represent a limited, but fundamental, set of guidelines that all tests which claim to measure linguistic knowledge (of any dialect) should be able to meet:

1. The test should be based on valid assumptions about language.
2. The test should be able to account for language variation.
3. The test should be based on a developmental model.
4. The results of the test should provide principled guidelines for language intervention.
5. The test should be able to provide an adequate description of some aspect of the child's knowledge of language.
6. The test should reflect the latest developments in linguistic theory.

Each criterion will be discussed in turn.

The Test Should Be Based on Valid Assumptions About Language

Before constructing a language evaluation tool, the test constructor at some point must ask the basic questions: What does it mean to know a language? Or, what does a speaker have to know before it can be concluded that he or she knows language A or B? Linguistic research has shown that to know a language involves (1) knowing the concepts that represent the objects, events, and relationships in the world; (2) knowing the linguistic forms that code these concepts; (3) knowing the set of rules (phonological, semantic, syntactic) that govern the possible combinations of forms; and (4) knowing the set of rules that govern the use of linguistic forms. If all or some of the assumptions about what it means to know a language are invalid, these underlying shortcomings will be reflected in the evaluation tool, and it will be incapable of adequately assessing language function.

The Utah Test of Language Development (UTLD) (Mecham, Jex, and Jones, 1969) is an example of a test that is based on several inadequate assumptions about what it means to know a language. More than half (53 percent) of the items included in the UTLD are extraneous to an assessment of a speaker's linguistic knowledge, in that they focus on academic, motor, or memory tasks, as opposed to tasks that assess knowledge of the basic components of language (i.e., semantics, syntax, pragmatics, and phonology). The numbers of these items, the tasks required, and descriptions for their nonlinguistic foci are presented in Table 2–2.

A speaker may know the basic rules underlying the grammatical, semantic, and pragmatic systems of his or her language yet not be able to complete successfully any of the tasks at his age level listed in Table 2–2. The inclusion of such tasks clearly indicates that many of the assumptions about linguistic knowledge which underlie the UTLD are invalid.

The Test Should Be Able to Account for Language Variation

Sociolinguistic research has shown that the forms of a language used to code concepts can vary as a function of age, sex, social class, ethnicity, and geographical region. Standard English, Black English, and Appalachian English are all varieties of the English language in which differences can be attributed to one or more of the factors just cited. Most assessment tools ignore language variation when specifying language concepts.

Table 2-2. Nonlinguistic Items in the Utah Test of Language Development

Item	Task	Task Type	Age Level (in years)	Description of Non-Li...
3	Mark with a pencil or crayon	motor	1–2	The ability to mark with a pencil or crayon is a n... example, a speaker whose hands are paralyzed will n... to use writing instruments effectively; however, he will be ... to speak normally if no paralysis affects the speech mechanism.
11	Repeat two digits	short-term memory	2–3	The relationship between the ability to recall digits and the ability to speak a language was not specified by the test authors. Thus, no framework is provided for interpreting a child's response to this item. It is possible, for example, for a child to be unable to recall two digits, in sequence, from memory, but yet exhibit normal linguistic behavior. The primary focus of a test of language development should be linguistic knowledge (i.e., semantic, pragmatic, syntactic, or phonological knowledge), not knowledge or related skills, such as sequential memory.
16	Repeat three digits	short-term memory	3–4	See Item 11.
19	Say a nursery rhyme from memory in the correct sequence	specific experience	3–4	A child between the ages of 3 and 4 (the expected age levels for successful completion of this item) could exhibit normal language development, but yet be unable to recite a nursery rhyme owing to lack of experience with this type of task. In order for a child to learn a nursery rhyme, someone in his home or school environment must value this skill and teach it to him. If a child is not exposed to rhymes, he will not learn them.
20	Copy a cross	perceptual motor	3–4	The ability to copy a cross is a perceptual motor skill. See also Item 3.
22	Repeat four digits	short-term memory	4–5	See Item 11.

Table continued on the following page

Table 2-2.   Nonlinguistic Items in the Utah Test of Language Development (continued)

Item	Task	Task Type	Age Level (in years)	Description of Non-Linguistic Focus
24	Repeat a twelve syllable sentence	short-term memory	4–5	See Item 11.
26	Copy a square	perceptual motor	5–6	See Items 3 and 20.
27	Print simple words	academic and motor	5–6	See Items 3 and 30.
29	Identify (by naming) a penny, nickel, and dime	specific experience	6–7	The ability to identify coins will be affected by the child's exposure to their correct names. A child with normal language development, but who has had limited or no opportunity to use coins, may respond incorrectly to this item.
30	Write numbers to the thirties	academic	6–7	This is an academic task. There are many illiterate people in the world who cannot write numbers to the thirties; however, they are competent speakers of a language.
32	Read words on preprimer level	academic	6–7	See Item 30.
33	Recite numbers from one to 50	academic	6–7	See Item 30.
34	Copy a diamond	perceptual motor	6–7	See Items 3 and 20.
36	Identify (by naming) a quarter, a half dollar, and a dollar	specific experience	7–8	See Item 29.
37	Repeat five digits	short-term memory	7–8	See Item 11.
38	Name the days of the week	long-term memory	7–8	This is a memory task which is formally taught in school. See also Item 11.

39	Repeat a 16 syllable sentence	short-term memory	8–10	See Item 11.
40	Write cursively with a pencil	academic and motor	8–10	See Items 3 and 30.
41	Rhyme words	metalinguistic	8–10	Rhyming words is a metalinguistic task that involves analysis of language on a conscious level. This task is emphasized, and in many cases learned in the school setting. The ability to rhyme requires a fairly high degree of awareness about the phonological shapes of words. It is possible that some children between the ages of 8 and 10 might not be very successful at rhyming words (especially if they are commanded to: "Tell me the name of an animal that rhymes with fair," p. 19, UTLD manual) but will be quite successful at speaking a language.
42	Repeat four digits reversed	short-term memory	8–10	See Item 11.
44	Repeat six digits reversed	short-term memory	10–15	See Item 11.
45	Repeat a 20 syllable sentence	short-term memory	10–15	See Item 11.
46	Repeat five digits reversed	short-term memory	10–15	See Item 11.
48	Repeat five mono-syllable words	short-term memory	10–15	See Item 11.
49	Repeat a difficult sentence from memory	short-term memory	10–15	See Item 11.
51	Answer questions regarding direction	specific experience	10–15	Many children between the ages of 10 and 15 will not have had the specific experience required to answer complex questions about compass points. Consider the following question from the UTLD manual (p. 21): "Suppose you are going *north*, then turn *left* again, then *right*, and then *right* again; what direction are you going now?" Many competent adult speakers will not be able to answer this question correctly.

For example, the GCS penalizes a testee who does not use the standard English code. This is true also for many other tests, including the UTLD, the Houston Test of Language Development (HTLD) (Crabtree, 1963), the Bankson Language Screening Test (BLST) (Bankson, 1978), and the DSS. In fact, the author of the DSS emphasizes that the procedure is "appropriate only for children learning standard American-English grammar" (Lee, 1974). Although this statement protects speakers of other dialects from having the forms characteristic of their dialects evaluated according to the DSS standard English norms, it also serves as a rationale for maintaining this unnecessary limitation. Studies of Black, Appalachian, and Puerto Rican English have described some of the features unique to these language varieties. Thus, it is possible to adapt a procedure so that it will be appropriate for examinees who speak nonstandard varieties of English. When adaptations are not provided, the title of the test should reflect the fact that it is appropriate only for a select group of speakers. For example, because of its focus the GCS should be called the Standard English Grammatic Closure Subtest. Such a title would specifically indicate that this test should not be used to evaluate the morphological systems of nonstandard speakers.

The realization that most language tests do not provide methods for handling dialect variation grows out of the erroneous notion that knowledge of a language involves knowing a particular variety of linguistic forms rather than knowing universal aspects of language. Valid assessment tools should have a universal perspective, that is, they should assess such universal concepts as negation, possession, causality, and plurality, with less focus on the specific forms that are used to code these concepts.

The Test Should Be Based on a Developmental Model

For an assessment tool to indicate whether a system is developing normally, it must provide a method of evaluating the order in which specific linguistic knowledge appears in a child's system. For example, studies of phonological acquisition have shown that stops are generally acquired before homorganic fricatives; thus it would be predicted that if a child can produce fricatives he or she should also be able to produce stops. Violations of expected patterns often provide evidence of deviant development.

In addition to considering the order in which knowledge is acquired, an assessment procedure should also be concerned about the age at which linguistic information is acquired. Studies have shown a fairly wide range of variation with respect to age of acquisition.

For example, the children Adam, Sarah, and Eve, discussed by Brown (1973), acquired the present progressive marker at ages 2 years 6 months, 2 years 10 months, and 1 year 9 months, respectively. Overall, the findings of the language acquisition research indicate a near invariant order with respect to the acquisition of linguistic knowledge; however, extensive variation in the age at which specific knowledge is acquired has been reported. A reliable statement regarding when a child is expected to exhibit certain linguistic information should be based on observations of language development in a fairly large number of children.

The Results of the Test Should Provide Principled Guidelines for Language Intervention

If the first guideline cannot be met, that is, if the fundamental assumptions underlying the tool are not valid, no basis will exist for developing principled intervention procedures. Consider, for example, the lack of direction that the PPVT provides for language intervention. Although the examiner can presumably calculate the testee's intelligence quotient, percentile score, and mental age, the results of the test do not provide any theoretically supported suggestions regarding which vocabulary items should be taught at different stages in a child's intervention program.

Although little is known about the details of lexical growth, research in language acquisition (e.g., Lahey and Bloom, 1977; Nelson, 1973) has shown that very young children use relational words (e.g., *more, all gone, no*), as well as substantive words (e.g., *dog, cat, man*) like those included in the PPVT. The former class of words code very important semantic notions in language and should be considered, therefore, when evaluating a child's lexicon. The lexicon, then, is not just a set of random words that can be easily depicted pictorially. What is acquired in a specific sequence is a set of forms that code meaning and when a child's vocabulary is not examined from this perspective, the results are not likely to provide an adequate direction for language intervention.

The Test Should Be Able to Provide an Adequate Description of Some Aspect of the Child's Knowledge of Language

Given the enormous complexity of language, it would be unrealistic for a test to attempt to evaluate in detail every aspect of a speaker's linguistic knowledge. An adequate test should have a clearly defined focus — that is, it should be specifically designed to assess the grammatical, semantic, or pragmatic systems or subcomponents within these systems. The inability of a tool to elicit the appropriate data for revealing a speaker's knowledge about at least one of the components of language generally indicates that false assumptions about the nature of language underlie its theoretical foundation. When the UTLD and HTLD are examined within the framework of this criterion, it can be seen that neither of these tools is capable of eliciting systematic information about a particular subsystem of language. Both tests contain an unfocused collection of items, many of which — as noted earlier — elicit behaviors that are totally unrelated to existing descriptions of linguistic knowledge.

The Test Should Reflect the Latest Developments in Linguistic Theory

The progress that has been made in language assessment in the 1970s and 1980s is very impressive. It is noteworthy, however, that some of the major advances have had almost no effect on the assessment of language in nonmainstream speakers. This observation is shown by the fact that many of the new tools that reflect the current foci on pragmatics and semantics are not appropriate for nonmainstream speakers. This shortcoming was openly acknowledged by Wiig (1982) in her pragmatics test, "Let's Talk Inventory for Adolescents," as follows:

> The item design presents a deliberate bias against a speaker who is not a representative of standard American English. This bias was dictated by the recognition that social-interpersonal communication acts differ as a function of language community. The inventory was designed to be appropriate for probing the ability to formulate and associate speech acts representative of speakers of standard American English.
>
> (Wiig 1982, p. 4)

Nearly all of the recently developed assessment devices that are appropriate for nonmainstream speakers focus only on linguistic form and not semantics or pragmatics (Vaughn-Cooke, 1984). These include the Screening Kit of Language Development (Bliss and Allen, 1983) and the Black English Sentence Scoring Technique (Nelson, 1983). The theoretical framework that guided the development of the Skold and the BESS is not current, for it ignores new developments in both pragmatics and semantics. Bloom (1971) presented evidence that showed convincingly that frameworks which focus only on form are inadequate and should be abandoned.

Language assessment tools for nonmainstream speakers have

lagged behind those for their mainstream counterparts because test constructors have generally failed to abandon the old, noncurrent form framework, even in the 1980s. Instead of assessing semantic and pragmatic knowledge, test constructors have been concerned with devising scoring systems that will give credit for nonmainstream forms (see in particular Nelson's Black English Sentence Scoring Technique). Unquestionably, such scoring systems are necessary, but they are not sufficient. What is needed are tools that have nonbiased scoring systems *and* the capacity to evaluate the pragmatic or the semantic dimensions of a nonmainstream speaker's language. Tools that do not exhibit these critical features are inadequate, and language assessment specialists need to be mindful of their limitations.

In conclusion, professionals who accept the important challenge of developing new language assessment devices for nonmainstream speakers should recognize the importance of knowing what is required to develop appropriate tools for these speakers. The guidelines discussed in this chapter specify some of the basic requirements. They can serve as a beginning point for those who wish to initiate test development.

ACKNOWLEDGMENTS

Research for this chapter was supported in part by NIH grant #RR08005. Portions of this paper appeared in Vaughn-Cooke, F. (1983). Improving language assessment in minority children. *ASHA, 25,* 29–34.

REFERENCES

Adler, S. (1971). Dialectical differences: Professional and clinical implications. *Journal of Speech and Hearing Disorders, 36,* 90–100.

Arnold, K. S., and Reed, L. (1976). The grammatic closure subtest of the ITPA: A comparative study of Black and White children. *Journal of Speech and Hearing Disorders, 41,* 477–485.

Bailey, D. B., and Harbin, G. L. (1980). *Nondiscriminatory evaluation. Exceptional Children, 46,* 590–595.

Bankson, N. (1977). *Bankson language screening test.* Baltimore: University Park Press.

Baratz, J. C. (1969a). Language and cognitive assessment of Negro children: Assumptions and research needs. *ASHA, 10,* 87–91.

Baratz, J. C. (1969b). Teaching reading in an urban Negro school system. In J. C. Baratz and R. W. Shuy (Eds.) *Teaching Black children to read.* Washington, DC: Center for Applied Linguistics.

Bergquist, C. C. (1982). A methodology for validating placement of children in exceptional child programs. *Exceptional Children, 49,* 269–270.

Bingham, V., and Ross, D. (1984). Letter to the chairperson of the Committee on the Status of Racial Minorities, American Speech, Language and Hearing Association.

Bliss, L. S., and Allen, D. V. (1983). *Screening kit of language development.* Baltimore: University Park Press.

Bloom, L. (1971). Why not pivot grammar? *Journal of Speech and Hearing Disorders, 36,* 40–50.

Brown, R. (1973) *A first language: The early stages.* Cambridge, MA: Harvard University Press.

Carrow, E. (1974). *The Carrow Elicited Language Inventory.* Austin: Learning Concepts.

Crabtree, M. (1963). *The Houston Test for language development. Part II,* Houston: Houston Test Co.

Daniel, J. L., and Scott, J. (1981). Language and communication skills. In G. Smitherman, (Ed.), *Black English and the education of Black children and youth.* Detroit: Harlo Press.

DeAvila, E., and Havassy, B. (1974, November–December). The testing of minority children — neo-Piagetian approach. *Today's Education,* 72–75.

Drew, C. J. (1973). Criterion-referenced and norm-referenced assessment of minority children. *Journal of School Psychology, 11,* 323–329.

Drumwright, A., Van Natta, P., Camp, B., Frankenburg, W., and Drexler, H. (1973). The Denver articulation screening exam. *Journal of Speech and Hearing Disorders, 38,* 3–14.

Duffy, J. B., Salvia, J., Tucker, J., and Ysseldyke, J. (1981). Nonbiased assessment: A need for operationalism. *Exceptional Children, 47,* 427–434.

Dunn, L. M., and Dunn, L. M. (1981). *Peabody picture vocabulary test — revised.* Circle Pines, MN: American Guidance Service.

Englemann, S., Ross, D., and Bingham, V. (1982). *Basic language concepts test.* Tigard, OR: C. C. Publications, Inc.

Evard, B. L., and McGrady, H. J. (1974). *Development of local language norms for Papago Indians, Mexican-Americans, Blacks, and Anglos.* Paper presented at the Annual Convention of the American Speech and Hearing Association, Las Vegas, NV.

Evard, B. L., and Sabers, D. L. (1974). *Development of local norms for Papago Indians, Mexican-Americans, Blacks, and Anglos for the Templin-Darley Tests of Articulation.* Paper presented at the Annual Convention of the American Speech and Hearing Association, Las Vegas, NV.

Evard, B. L., and Sabers, D. L. (1979). Speech and language testing with distinct ethnic-racial groups: A survey of procedures for improving validity. *Journal of Speech and Hearing Disorders, 44,* 271–281.

Hemingway, B. L., Montague, J. C., and Bradley, R. H. (1981). Preliminary data on revision of a sentence repetition test for language screening with Black first grade children. *Language, Speech, and Hearing Services in the Schools, 12,* 153–159.

Kaimowitz, G., and Lewis, K. (1979). Martin Luther King Junior Elementary School Children, et al. vs. The Michigan Board of Education, the Michigan Superintendent of Public Instruction, et al. Second Amended Complaint, Preliminary Statement. Detroit, MI.

Kirk, S., McCarthy, J., and Kirk, W. (1968). *Illinois Test of Psycholinguistic*

Abilities. Urbana, IL: University of Illinois Press.

Lahey, M., and Bloom, L. (1977). Planning a first lexicon: Which words to teach first. *Journal of Speech and Hearing Disorders, 42,* 340–350.

Larson, R., and Olson, L. (1963). A method of identifying culturally deprived kindergarten children. *Exceptional Children, 29,* 130–134.

Lee, L. (1974). *Developmental sentence analysis.* Evanston, IL: Northwestern University Press.

Leonard, L. B., Perozzi, J., Prutting, C. S., and Berkeley, R. K. (1978). Nonstandard approaches to the assessment of language behaviors. *ASHA, 20,* 371–379.

Leonard, L. B., and Weiss, A. L. (1983). Application of nonstandardized assessment procedures to diverse linguistic populations. *Topics in Language Disorders, 3,* 35–45.

Lively-Weiss, M. A., and Koller, D. E. (1973). Selected language characteristics of middle-class and inner-city children. *Journal of Communication Disorders, 6,* 303–314.

McConnell, F., Horton, K., and Smith, B. (1969, April). Language Development and Cultural Disadvantagement. *Exceptional Children, 35,* 597–606.

Mecham, J., Jex, J., and Jones, J. (1969). *Utah test of language development.* Salt Lake City: Communication Research Associates.

Mercer, J. R., (1983). Issues in the diagnosis of language disorders in students whose primary language is not English. *Topics in Language Disorders, 3,* 46–56.

Nelson, K. (1973). Structure and Strategy in Learning to Talk. *Monographs of the Society for Research in Child Development 38* (No. 149).

Nelson, N. (1976). *Dialect differences in language samples gathered from Black preschoolers: Interviewer effects and measurement procedures.* Paper presented at the American Speech and Hearing Association Convention, Houston.

Nelson, N. (1983). *Black English Sentence Scoring: A tool for nonbiased assessment.* Paper presented at the annual convention of the American Speech-Language-Hearing Association, Cincinnati, OH.

Politzer, R. L., Hoover, M. R., and Brown, D. (1974). A test of proficiency in Black standard and nonstandard speech. *TESOL Quarterly, 8,* 27–35.

Reveron, W. W. (1983). *Language assessment of Black children: The state of the art.* Paper presented at the Fifth Annual Conference of the National Black Association for Speech, Language and Hearing, Washington, DC.

Rychman, D. B. (1967). A comparison of information processing abilities of middle- and lower-class Negro kindergarten boys. *Exceptional Children, 33,* 545–552.

Seymour, H. N., and Miller-Jones, D. (1981). Language and cognitive assessment of Black children. *Speech and language: Advances in basic research and practice, 6,* 203–263.

Shuy, R., and Staton, J. (1982). Assessing oral language ability in children. In P. Dickson (Ed.), *The language of children reared in poverty.* New York: Academic Press.

Smith, H. W., and May, W. T. (1967). Influence of the examiner on the ITPA scores of Negro children. *Psychological Reports, 20,* 499–502.

Stephenson, B. L., and Gay, W. O. (1972). Psycholinguistic abilities of Black and White children from four SES levels. *Exceptional Children, 36,* 705–709.

Africa and the diaspora. Paper presented at the First World Congress on Communication in Africa and the Diaspora, Nairobi, Kenya.

Taylor, O. T., and Payne, K. T. (1983). Culturally valid testing: A proactive approach. *Topics in Language Disorders, 3,* 1–7.

Vaughn-Cooke, A. F. (1979). Evaluating language assessment procedures: An examination of linguistic guidelines and Public Law 94-142 guidelines. In J. E. Alatis and R. Tucker (Eds.), *Language and public life: Proceedings of the Thirtieth Annual Georgetown University Roundtable,* Washington, DC.

Vaughn-Cooke, A. F. (1980). Evaluating the language of Black English speakers: Implications of the Ann Arbor decision. In M. F. Whiteman (Ed.), *Reactions to Ann Arbor: Vernacular Black English and education.* Washington, DC: Center for Applied Linguistics.

Vaughn-Cooke, A. F. (1984, September). *Theoretical frameworks and language assessment.* Paper presented at the National Symposium on Concerns for Minority Groups in Communication Disorders, Vanderbilt University.

Weiner, P. S., and Hoock, W. C. (1973). The standardization of tests: Criteria and criticisms. *Journal of Speech and Hearing Research, 16,* 616–626.

Wiig, E. (1982). *Let's talk inventory for adolescents.* Columbus: Charles E. Merrill Publishing Co.

Williams, R. L. (1972). *The BITCH-100: A culture specific test.* St. Louis, MO: Williams and Associates.

Williams, R. L. (1970). Danger: Testing and dehumanizing Black children. *Clinical Child Psychology Newsletter, 9* (1), 5–6.

Wolfram, W. A. (1983). Test interpretation and sociolinguistic differences. *Topics in Language Disorders, 3,* 21–34.

Wolfram, W. A., Williams, R., and Taylor, O. (1972). *Some predicted dialect interference in select language development tests.* Short course presented at the Annual Convention of the American Speech-Language and Hearing Association, Rockville, MD.

Ysseldyke, J. E., and Regan, R. R. (1980). Nondiscriminatory assessment: A formative model. *Exceptional Children, 46,* 465–466.

Chapter 3

Nonstandardized Approaches to Speech and Language Assessment

Audrey L. Holland and Margaret Forbes

Systematic field observation is used extensively by social and behavioral scientists in studying many aspects of human interaction. As Chapter 1 suggests, the rich language variation of differing cultural groups can be studied most productively using the techniques of ethnographic analysis. It is itself an excellent example of bias that when the tools of systematic field observation are applied to clinical speech and language assessment, they become known as "nonstandard" approaches. The underlying assumption of that peculiar bit of semantics is, of course, that the "real" way to assess speech and language behavior is through formal and standard testing procedures. We would quarrel with this assumption, both for speech and language disordered individuals who differ linguistically and culturally from mainstream white middle class Americans and for those who are part of that mainstream. To derive a complete picture of an individual's ability to use speech and language, and to comprehend the speech and language of others, observation in natural contexts is a necessity. Furthermore, if the investigator is trying to become a sensitive clinician, observation provides a source of information about a particular individual that can only be guessed at from standard assessments or from watching the completion of clinical assignments across a table. Standard assessment procedures are, needless to say, useful for providing baselines against which progress can be charted, for communicating briefly and succinctly with other professionals, for comparing performance of a single person to the normative sample, and so forth. Nevertheless, standardized measures alone fail to present a complete picture of a given person's ability to use and comprehend language and must be augmented by so-called "non-standard" procedures.

This chapter describes some ways to sample natural and everyday speech and language behaviors. Some of these procedures are more natural and "everyday" than others, and guidelines will be suggested for how and when to use them. Simply gathering language samples in and of itself is not a virtue, however; the language samples must be analyzed. Therefore, some forms of analysis are described that might be particularly useful. Because probe techniques are also useful diagnostically, they too will be described briefly. Finally, it is our belief that structured parent-family interviewing is a valuable procedure for nonstandard assessment. We describe a few such procedures to conclude this chapter.

The term "nonstandard assessment" will not be used further here. Rather, we will replace that controversial term with more descriptive words such as observing, sampling, probing language behavior, and analyzing the language samples that result. Whenever possible, we will draw our examples and our data from language studies of children and adults who are not middle class, white, American English speakers. However, we remain committed to the belief that most of the comments we make apply equally strongly to studying disordered language in that population as well.

SAMPLING SPONTANEOUS LANGUAGE

A spontaneous language sample is collected for the purpose of examining a person's usual language. To be useful, the sample must represent the client's ordinary use of language in everyday communicative situations.

To most speech and language clinicians, "spontaneous speech" is synonymous with asking a child or adult to describe a picture or with engaging him or her in a brief conversation. Comparisons are then made between this "more natural" speech and the results of formal language tests. The comparisons usually take the form of holistic judgments about whether the observed behavior is predictable from the test performance.

General Problems. A number of problems arise with the use of clinician-client interaction picture description as the sole free speech-language base. For the most part, these problems are similar, whether the clinician is obtaining spontaneous language samples from speakers of standard or nonstandard English, but certain special considerations must be kept in mind with speakers of nonstandard English, especially if the examiner's usual language is standard English and he or she differs culturally from the client. This variable of cultural mismatch can greatly complicate the issue. No direct information is available on language disordered adults from cultural and racial minority groups. Work with children, however, suggests that the mismatch of white examiner–black child can result in potentially misleading information. A number of authors have addressed this issue (Hall and Nagy, 1981; Johnson, 1974; Seymour and Miller-Jones, 1981). A credible summary of concerns over these mismatches indicates that not only do dialectal variations create some problems but also cross-cultural language samples are even less likely to reflect the speaker's proficiency than samples collected when culture and dialect are colliding.

Often speakers of nonstandard English are self-conscious about the difference in their language. They respond to this knowledge in a variety of ways. For example, some may feel that their form of language is somehow "inferior" and may therefore speak only briefly and with restraint, some may try to use "standard" English, in which they are less competent, and others may respond with anger or defensiveness. In none of these instances is the resulting language sample representative of normal use.

A clinician must be particularly sensitive to his or her own and the client's nonverbal behavior. The client's nonverbal behavior, acquired in a culture different from the examiner's, may be unfamiliar to the examiner. Unless he or she is especially vigilant, the examiner may miss nonverbal clues betraying discomfort, shyness, anger, and other emotions that the client is unable or unwilling to verbalize. All such feelings may interfere with a client's ability to speak in his or her usual way. The examiner must also be aware of his or her own nonverbal behavior and most especially of its effects on the client. The unwary clinician may inadvertently communicate negative judgments or attitudes he or she does not feel or intend to convey. A client who fears or expects such judgments may read them into the clinician's actions or expressions irrespective of what the clinician does. The best a clinician can do under such circumstances is to try to identify and then to empathize with the client's feelings and to convey caring and supportiveness both verbally and nonverbally. An examiner whom a client perceives as judgmental, cold, or condescending will have little success in eliciting normal language, even if he or she is not intentionally projecting such attitudes. A comfortable nonverbal rapport is as important as a comfortable setting for collecting a spontaneous language sample representative of a child's normal performance. Although these considerations are also important in collecting language samples from speakers of standard English, they are accentuated when a standard English speaker is evaluating the language of someone who speaks nonstandard English. The sensitive examiner should be aware that such a client is likely to feel quite vulnerable and should make every effort to ensure that the client feels comfortable and accepted.

An attractive solution to these problems is to have an examiner whose language and cultural milieu are similar to those of the person being evaluated. Unfortunately, this is often impossible, but the aware examiner can manipulate some of the situational factors that strongly affect the quality of language sample and thus make the process less strange and frightening.

Situational Factors. Most important among the situational factors that can affect the representativeness of a person's performance during the collection of a language sample are the following: (1) rapport between the client and the examiner, (2) the setting, (3) the stimuli, and (4) the size of the sample. The clinician must be aware of the effect of these factors and control them to the best of his or her ability.

The first factor, rapport between examinee and examiner, is greatly influenced by the examiner's sensitivity to the individual client. Different listeners also appear to produce different language behaviors (Olswang and Carpenter, 1978). However benign the clinical setting and however careful the clinician is who initially assesses a given client, that clinician is by definition a stranger, and the language sample gathered may have limited generalizability to the child's or adult's more familiar world. As an example from the adult literature, Helmick, Watamori, and Palmer (1976) compared performances on the Porch Index of Communicative Ability (PICA) with family members' estimates of language adequacy for a sample of adult aphasic patients. Because the estimates failed to correlate significantly, and because PICA scores indicated more severe language problems than family members had estimated, Helmick and associates concluded that families overestimated their aphasic family members' abilities. Holland (1976) argued that although the discrepancy might well be valid, it was equally possible that PICA erred by underestimating language performance at home. That this interpretation did not occur to the authors further suggests that test behavior and language samples taken in the clinic are possibly more consonant than is clinic language and language used beyond its doors. The nonverbal behavior mentioned previously is especially important here, as the person who perceives warmth and acceptance from the examiner at the nonverbal level is likely to feel more relaxed and comfortable.

This is only a first step, however. In addition to putting the person at ease, the clinician must establish rapport in such a way that the client is willing to talk. First, especially with children, the clinician needs to adjust his or her own communicative behavior to the client's developmental level, making certain that the client is able to comprehend and relate to what is said to him or her. Miller (1981) suggests that a clinician wishing to encourage a child to talk should be "interested without being pushy." Open-ended questions such as "what happened next?" elicit talking better than closed questions or commands. Reticent children often respond well to the examiner's saying very little for 5 minutes after the initial friendly greeting. These few minutes can be a companionable time between the child and examiner and can be spent in parallel play, with the examiner addressing any talking to the toys rather than the child, or in interactive play, in which the child is invited but not commanded to participate. After this "warm-up" time, the child is likely to begin verbalizing on his or her own, and the examiner can continue to provide interested, supportive encouragement.

Although the clinician's interaction with an adult is likely to be entirely verbal, without the use of toys or periods of not talking, the principle of being interested but not pushy still applies. In general, a warm, accepting, nondemanding clinician has the best chance of developing good rapport with the client and thus facilitating a representative language sample.

The second situational factor, the setting, can also be used to help ensure a representative language sample. For example, the clinical environment itself appears to have a limiting effect on the language sample. Scott and Taylor (1978), studying normal children, showed them to produce significantly longer utterances at home than in the clinic. Furthermore, clinic language sampling was "conducive to the description of ongoing and imminent activity, while home sampling stimulated substantially higher frequencies of past tense and modal verb forms, complex utterances and questions." Kramer, James, and Saxman (1979) studied children who had been referred to a speech clinic for language disorders. They found home language samples yielded longer mean lengths of utterance (MLUs) and higher estimated language ages on the Developmental Sentence Scoring (DSS) than did samples obtained in the clinic. For these reasons, it is desirable to collect language samples for a given client in several different familiar settings. When this is possible, the examiner can use the setting to enhance the client's comfort and hence the quality of the language sample.

A simple way to ease the discomfort of a client who feels self-conscious about his or her language is to arrange for the first sample to be collected in a place where he or she is at ease, such as the client's own home. With a child, the first sample might best be collected while the child engages in spontaneous play with the mother or another child, with the examiner (and a tape recorder) present in only a minor role. A child who gradually becomes accustomed to having his or her talking tape-recorded with an unknown examiner in the room is less likely to be intimidated by the evaluation process than one who is immediately asked to perform in an unfamiliar place with an unknown person. A good way to find out where a particular child might feel at ease is to ask the child's family or teachers prior to the evaluation. An adult client can be asked where she or she would feel most comfortable, or the clinician may merely arrange a first meeting at the client's home.

We recognize that this is the ideal, and we further recognize that the ideal is seldom practical in clinical work. Nevertheless, rather than throw up our hands or relegate these beliefs about the importance of setting to the more cushy world of language research, the creative clinician should attempt to approximate the principles in the clinic. For example, the first in-clinic sample can be collected in the presence of familiar people (families in the case of adults, parents in the case of children) in the clinic's most comfortable setting, rather than across a desk or play table. The point is to take advantage of whatever features of a given clinic maximize a homey feel.

A third situational variable the examiner can manipulate is the choice of stimuli used to elicit the sample. When a clinician has developed good rapport with a client in a comfortable setting, the client may be ready to talk. But unless the stimuli are interesting and relevant, there might be little reason to talk. "Stimuli" in this context may merely be the subject matter the clinician chooses to introduce if the client runs out of ideas of what to talk about. Stimuli may also include objects or, for children, toys to facilitate conversational interaction between the client and the clinician. Although it is certainly desirable for the client to talk more than the clinician, a language sample should reflect the client's normal language as it is used to communicate with another person — as opposed to an artificial use of language, such as describing a picture or object to a clinician who already knows what it looks like. A "spontaneous sample"

consisting of description of a picture or object is a highly questionable example of a person's normal use of language. Labov (1976) cau-
tioned investigators long ago about the differences inherent in language samples obtained when the speaker is, in effect, "commanded
to talk" and the sample that results from true free expression (i.e.,
spontaneous speech).

Even within the confines of being commanded to talk, there are
ways superior to picture description for "freeing" the speaker a bit.
Among them are using story retell techniques and using good questions. In an unpublished study, Holland compared performances of
children who were very well known to her (black, white, and bilingual Japanese-English speaking playmates of her own children,
then ages 8 and 10). Two language elicitation tasks were compared
in a familiar setting. For one task, the children were given the verbal expression subtest of the ITPA (i.e., "Tell me everything you can
about this button"). For the second, each child was asked to "tell me
about the scariest thing that ever happened to you." Samples were
compared on grammatical complexity, length, MLU, and other aspects. In no instance was any child's performance on the "scary experience" task predictable from the ITPA task, and in all instances the
ITPA test predicted shorter length, shorter MLU, and less complex
grammar.

For a child, prior to the evaluation, an examiner can prepare for
the language sampling session by discussing the child's interests
and enthusiasms with his or her parents and teachers. Bloom and
Lahey (1978) found that children tend to produce a greater number
and variety of language behaviors when the conversation revolves
around a concrete activity, such as construction, science experi-
ments, or art projects, and the child just talks about the activities
rather than being specifically questioned about them. Lee (1974)
found that having very young children describe pictures evoked less
spontaneous speech than playing with toys. Bloom and Lahey point
out that children often merely label pictures, thus producing unsatisfactory language samples. Older children, on the other hand, talk
more about pictures. Longhurst and File (1977) and others have
found that, on the whole, more language and more complex language are elicited in unstructured than in structured situations.
With adults the clinician needs to be attuned to what is interesting
to the client, as well what he or she finds comfortable to talk about.

The fourth situational factor the clinician can manipulate is the
length of the sample, in terms of either time or number of utterances. No agreement has yet been reached about the minimum
length of a sample, and so the clinician is left to make a judgment. To

calculate the MLU, at least 50 utterances are needed, and Tyack and Gottsleben (1974) suggest a minimum of 50 to 100 utterances for a sample to be used for a clinical analysis. For children with limited repertoires, 50 utterances appear to be sufficient. For adults, partly because what constitutes a single utterance is so difficult to define, transcriptions of 50 utterances appear to be the minimum. Fortunately, a larger sample can be obtained rather rapidly (in about 5 to 10 minutes) for all but those with the most severe language problems. In terms of time, Bloom and Lahey (1978) suggest at least one half hour of specific observation, preferably in more than one setting on more than one day.

Time sampling problems were addressed in developing the procedure for systematic observation of interactive communicative behavior that was used with aphasic adults to validate Holland's measure of Communicative Abilities in Daily Living (CADL) (1980). Once features to be observed were defined, the experimental solution to determining a valid length of observation was simply to record a very long sample (in this case 4 hours), score the sample in consecutive 15 minute segments and note when no new, but only redundant, information appeared on the scoring sheet. It is of interest that 90 percent of the new information (defined according the categories used) appeared within the first 25 or 30 minutes, and after 60 minutes all features of concern were merely redundant. Therefore, we feel confident that a sample of 30 minutes in length, when free field observation is the milieu, is sufficient. For more constrained circumstances, as 15 minute observation is probably likely to tell the clinician enough. For a more complete description of procedures used to observe aphasic patients in their natural surroundings and the richness of such observations, see Holland (1982).

The foregoing criticisms of the procedures most often used in clinical settings can be met in a number of relatively simple ways. First, as we have already noted, to obtain a valid sample of speech and language behavior in a clinic is difficult because of setting. Particularly in the case of children, it is mandatory that clinical interaction samples are gathered with more than one interactant whenever possible. It is strongly urged that the interactants include individuals who have differing interactional histories with the child. For example, a parent-child sample is paramount, and it should be compared with the clinician-child sample. A child-child sample is also highly desirable. One possible solution to the setting problem is to observe the child at home. A more easily available alternative might be to send the parent home with a tape recorder, to be used to record brief interactions in the home.

It is reasonable to expect that adults with language disorders might show less variation than children do as a function of auditor and setting. Nevertheless, the possibility that they might show more variation exists. As a absolute minimum, family members should be observed in brief interaction and should also be asked, along with the language disordered adult, to judge and comment on the typicality of the speech sampled in interaction with the clinician. It is our practice simply to inquire if we are easy to talk to, or hard to, or somewhere in between, and why.

Second, it is important to recognize that a picture description can never be substituted for a free sample. A commanded sample is very useful because it can be analyzed efficiently, using some techniques to be described later in this chapter. But it is simply not a sample of spontaneous speech, and this difference must be recognized.

ANALYZING SPONTANEOUS SPEECH

It is obvious that the quality of a sample of spontaneous language depends to a great extend on the clinical skill and judgment of the examiner. No hard and fast rules apply. The same kind of judgment must be exercised in analyzing the sample once it is collected. Many different kinds of analysis exist, and the clinician must select those that will reveal the most information about the particular client being evaluated.

A variety of analyses are possible for spontaneous language samples, and as with the other aspects of language evaluation, particular care must be taken in analyzing the language of a speaker of nonstandard English. Once the examiner has determined that a client's usual language is a nonstandard form of English, what should be used as a basis of comparison to determine whether or not the client's language shows evidence of delay or other disorder becomes problematical. It is conceivable that a clinician can compare a client's language with that of other speakers of his or her own dialect. If such a strategy is undertaken, several difficulties may arise. Unless the clinician is a speaker of the client's dialect, she may well be unfamiliar with the correct forms or mistaken in her concept of them. She may therefore err in judgments of whether or not the client is using correct forms as they are normally used by speakers of a given dialect. Furthermore, for a child, there are no norms for the age of acquisition of nonstandard forms, making it difficult to determine whether the child's language use is delayed in comparison with his or her peers.

A productive method of analyzing the sample might be to evaluate the forms that occur both in the child's dialect and in standard English. A drawback to this method is that the child's language difficulties may be with forms that do not overlap with those of standard English, and his or her language problem may be overlooked. In addition, it is often a problem to determine which forms in a particular child's dialect are similar to those in standard English. Thus, although it is important to perform some analysis of form, it should be realized that considerable doubt and imprecision are inherent in such an analysis of nonstandard English, and analyses of form alone are insufficient bases for judging a person's language competence.

Analyzing semantic and pragmatic aspects of language in addition to structural aspects is even more critical with speakers of nonstandard English than it is with speakers of standard English. Because standard and nonstandard English differ in other ways as well, analysis of structure alone provides a highly unreliable picture of the client as a communicator.

Some aspects of language are relatively independent of the speaker's dialect, and it is useful to assess these in any client, but especially in a speaker of nonstandard English. Several relatively new computerized language analyses provide information about such aspects of language as MLU, number of bound morphemes, type token ratio (TTR), turn taking, and so forth. Other analyses address more traditional structural aspects of language. A selected group of useful analyses is described briefly here. Many more systems for analyzing language samples exist, and more are in the process of being developed. No one system is applicable to all clients. The clinician must learn as much as possible about the many kinds of analysis to be able to choose appropriately.

LARSP (Language Assessment, Remediation, and Screening Procedure (Crystal, 1979; Crystal, Fletcher, and Garman, 1976). The method devised by Crystal and associates for assessing free speech samples is primarily concerned with a structural analysis of syntax. It is based on the grammar of English written by Quirk, Greenbaum, Leech, and Svartvik (1972), itself a descriptive rather than an explanatory grammar. The system developed by Quirk and colleagues recognizes descriptive levels of sentence (major and minor), clause (phrase structure components), and word structure (morphology) and finally some functional components (statements, commands, questions, and explanations). Crystal and associates have essentially formalized and developed a systematic analysis form that allows the clinician to describe a sample of spontaneous speech in relation to the grammar of Quirk and colleagues. In the 1976 book and in subsequent writings, Crystal explains the method of coding speech samples and provides convincing data regarding the usefulness of the system in analyzing the emerging grammars of children with language disorders.

Although Crystal suggests that the system is applicable to linguistic description of aphasic adults, he has provided very little data. Two studies, those of Kearns and Simmons (1983) and Penn (1983), corroborate Crystal's claims. Penn used the system successfully to differentiate among three syntactical patterns of aphasia, giving credence to the system's validity. It is not our intent to describe in detail the method of scoring; for a complete description, it is critical to read Crystal's writings very carefully. Nevertheless, we believe LARSP is an important, potentially powerful, and very useful system for analyzing spontaneous speech. It has the additional advantage of providing a common language for clinicians to use in comparing samples of patients at more than one center.

Systematic Analysis of Language Samples (SALT) (Miller And Chapman, 1983). SALT is a computerized system for analyzing language samples along a number of traditional and useful dimensions, such as MLU, TTR, utterances per minute, and so forth. To have such features computerized is at least time-saving and reliable. However, the main advantages of the SALT system are its innovative features, such as measures of turn taking and speaker floor time, and its flexibility. SALT allows the user to search a transcript, prepared according to the manual and entered into a microcomputer, for a variety of preselected features. For example, all of the "mental words" in a transcript can be listed; or all of the conjunctions that provide an indirect measure of syntactical complexity can be listed. Some analyses are provided by Miller and Chapman, but users also have options that allow them to search transcripts for features that are of particular interest. Furthermore, transcripts can be coded in a number of ways that allow the user to highlight important aspects of language. For example, although it was devised initially as a way to analyze children's language, we have modified the SALT system so that at present it accommodates spontaneous speech by aphasic patients as well (Holland et al., 1985). A final SALT feature that is particularly useful for adult language is that SALT automatically provides data on all speakers involved in an interaction, if those speakers are identified by the person entering the transcript. We have so very little information available on adult normal speakers, particularly in conversational interaction, that this is indeed a boon. Using this kind of analysis, it is likely that we can investigate a number of features that will tell us about normal as well as abnormal speech.

As is true for all forms of language analysis regardless of

whether they are computerized or not, SALT requires the user to transcribe the sample. In the case of SALT, this transcription must be coded before entry into the computer. There is little doubt that both transcription and coding are time-consuming. However, we use SALT regularly, and our estimate is that if we were to perform the analyses we do on a 5 minute sample of aphasic–nonaphasic conversation "by hand," it would consume approximately 40 hours. A SALT analysis takes less than 6 hours.

The foregoing examples do not begin to exhaust the presently available computerized systems for the analysis of spontaneous language. We have highlighted these only because they are familiar to us.

PROBE TECHNIQUES

Analysis of spontaneous language production is fundamental to understanding language development and language disorders. However, the clinician must also be concerned with assessing how a person deals with the acquisition of new material and comprehends the speech of others. For these purposes, simply listening to and analyzing production is insufficient. Because these are critical clinical concerns, they partially explain the popularity of formal language tests.

Probe techniques for use in natural speech and language settings are also available for making such assessments systematically. Most of them derive from methods employed by psycholinguists to study specific aspects of children's acquisition of language, and as a result these methods are more widely applied to children's than to adults' language. Therefore, in the examples to follow, the speech of children will be highlighted. However, only the clinician's resourcefulness limits both the variety of features for which these procedures can be adapted and the types of language problems to which they can be applied.

Researchers such as Brown (1958), Nelson (1982), Leonard, Schwartz, Morris, and Chapman (1981), and MacWhinney (1982) have developed a simple way to get at children's assimilation of new items, a matter of obvious importance in assessing the likelihood of progress in treatment. The basic paradigm is always the same. In the context of free play, the child is shown a new object or activity and then the experimenter presents the child with a new word for this concept and assesses the child's ability to use this new word.

Learning New Words. Learning new words, chosen to exemplify a particular phonological aspect, might be used to assess the ease with which a child having a particular phonological problem can acquire the requisite pattern. For example, exotic and unfamiliar objects might be arbitrarily labeled with /s/ cluster names for a child who demonstrates /s/ cluster problems. His ability to repeat and to produce these new names (smalk, sporn, skeester, and so forth) is assessed in play situations. This new word paradigm can be used to assess a host of other abilities, such as lexical concepts, ability to structure semantic fields, and ability to extract meaning from context. As an example of the latter, here is an instance of co-occurrence frame learning. The clinician can point to a doll and call it "Ged" or "a ged." In the case of "Ged," the word is to be construed as a proper noun; in the case of "a ged," it is a common noun. For whatever purposes such new words are used, once a child has learned the new form, learning can be tested on subsequent days in a variant of Berko's procedure (1958). For example, the child learns on the first day to call a garlic press a "wug." On subsequent days he or she can be presented with two garlic presses and asked, "What are these?" In this way, the spontaneous production of plurals (in this case) or other forms can be assessed.

Responses to communicative probes can be observed. Although they do not constitute new structures, communicative probes allow clinicians to assess problems in pragmatic functioning. Here are a few examples: if the clinician is interested in assessing the ability to provide requests for clarification, Gallagher and Darnton (1978) and Newhoff, Tonkovich, Schwartz, and Burgess (1982) have described a useful approach, the former used effectively with children, the latter with adults who are aphasic. Several times during a spontaneous interaction, the clinician responds to a client's statement by simply saying, "What?" Such requests for clarification permit assessment of a variety of repairs.

In a different pragmatic vein, the study of responses to comments about performance or some personal aspect may inform us not only about communicative functioning but also about self-concept. For example, systematic inclusion in a free speech situation of comments such as "That's a pretty dress you have on" can be used as probes to check reactions to praise.

Comprehension. Probe techniques are most familiar to clinicians as ways to assess comprehension of language. Syntactic and semantic complexity and the ability to respond to questions and to commands of varying length have long been used to assess features of language comprehension. In fact, without including some of these probe techniques, the ability to comprehend can only be inferred, and it is limited merely to the exemplars that occur in spontaneous interaction.

A particularly fruitful new technique for studying sentence comprehension in children, across languages, has been developed over the past few years by MacWhinney, Bates, and their colleagues. It is intriguing to consider the use of their approaches across dialects as well. The work of these investigators has led to the formulation of a "competition model" for sentence comprehension. The basic technique is that of sentence enactment. Two toys are placed in front of the child — one horse and one cow. The child listens to a sentence such as "The horse pushes the cow" or "Pushes the horse the cow" and is asked to move the toys to show what happened. Bates, McNew, MacWhinney, Devescovi, and Smith (1982) and MacWhinney, Bates, and Kliegl (1984) have been able to obtain data from children as young as 2 years 4 months using the procedure and have recently begun extending the work to adults with aphasia in a cross-language study. Word order, agreement, and juncture can be varied systematically.

The foregoing merely hints at the vast possibilities of incorporating systematic probe techniques into assessment procedures. It is apparent that such techniques can be incorporated into spontaneous language interactions. Rather than creating "tests" of these and similar phenomena, we believe their systematic incorporation into spontaneous interactions is the route of choice. In that way, they share the advantage of naturalness with the spontaneous sample itself.

SYSTEMATIC INTERVIEW AS A FORM OF ASSESSMENT

We have previously alluded to the necessity of relying on clients themselves and on parents to give us information about the validity of the language samples we have been collecting. It is important to conclude this chapter by taking this concept one step further, that is, to discuss the advantages of systematic interviews as a source of data for language assessment. The power inherent in simply *asking* informants has never been fully appreciated by speech-language pathologists, although formalized approaches to asking appear to be gaining some credence as statistical techniques for evaluating the reliability and validity of such procedures are being applied to them. Particularly in the case of potential dialect and cultural mismatch between client and clinician, they appear to have a special potency. For example, if the clinician is truly unsure about whether or not a given speaker has a language problem or has speech that is within cultural expectations for his or her age and milieu, the clinician would do very well indeed to ask a few speakers of the dialect what they think about the person's speech and language.

But there are general problems that lend themselves very well to the use of more systematic interviewing about a client's language. Among them are the assessment of very young children, in which a slice of language observed by a clinician might not be nearly as representative or as valid as a parent's assessment of the child's performance, particularly if that assessment is guided by carefully constructed interview questions. Another example is gaining information about a poststroke aphasic patient's pretraumatic communicative abilities and style, so that appropriate treatment can be planned and enhanced. Often the best source of such information is the family rather than the patient, whose language deficit itself could interfere with the assessment.

One excellent interview protocol for parents of young children has been developed by Bretherton, Snyder, and colleagues (Bretherton and Beeghly, 1982; Snyder, Bates and Bretherton, 1981). This protocol has been demonstrated to correlate well with extensive language samples taken of the same children (Bretherton, McNew, Snyder, and Bates, 1983). Less well tested, but quite promising, is a communication assessment procedure developed by Ylvisaker (1983) for use with children between the ages of 6 and 24 months. This questionnaire looks not only at language but also at a number of developmental domains that are related to language acquisition. Rather than an interview procedure, this questionnaire is filled in by parents, and they are given specific tasks to perform with their children to help them answer some of the questions.

A less formal but insightful procedure for parent interviews is used by Liebergott (personal communication) in her longitudinal study of premature infants. Liebergott simply requires parents in that study to keep extensive diaries of their children's developing vocabularies, which are shared with the investigators at specified times over the course of development. This procedure would be extremely simple to use in clinical as well as research environments, and it could provide an altogether different sample for analysis by clinicians.

Only a few questionnaires and interview protocols have been developed for adults, and none are in widespread use. Nevertheless, it is likely that such procedures would be very helpful in assessment of language impaired adults as well. Swindell, Pashek, and Holland (1982) developed a questionnaire for assessing pretraumatic communicative style of aphasic patients. Spouses served as informants. The questionnaire was validated using a sample of nonaphasic couples who completed the questionnaire both for themselves and for their spouses; good agreement was shown.

The use of interviews is an area in which much more remains to be done. Nevertheless, it is likely that the future will see more such techniques that capitalize on the experience and observation powers of individuals who have long-term contact with the child or adult in question. They appear to have general applicability, but in their use in situations of cultural mismatch, they could be particularly formidable.

CONCLUSIONS

In this chapter, we have attempted to provide some guidelines for gathering and analyzing spontaneous speech samples, for using probe techniques, and for invoking systematic interviewing procedures in the assessment of speech and language. Our bias has probably been evident throughout, but if it has remained obscure, we now wish to remedy that situation. We believe that the techniques from the domain we have described here are perhaps the most important tools that speech-language pathologists possess for assessing speech and language behaviors. If they are regarded as having more specialized use in situations of cultural mismatch between disordered individuals and those who assess them, then that is to the advantage of the mismatched themselves, and to the disadvantage of culturally similar clients and clinicians. Far from considering these approaches to be "nonstandard," we think of them as *the* standard and advocate that others adopt such a stance as well.

ACKNOWLEDGMENTS

Preparation of this manuscript has been supported by two research grants: NS17495-03 and G008300010, Audrey L. Holland, principal investigator. The authors acknowledge the extensive contributions to their thinking that have been provided by Brian MacWhinney.

REFERENCES

Bates, E., McNew, S., MacWhinney, B., Devescovi, A., and Smith, S. (1982). Functional constraints on sentence processing: A cross-linguistic study.

Cognition, 11, 245–299.

Berko, J. (1958). The child's learning of English morphology. *Word, 14,* 150–177.

Bloom, L., and Lahey, M. (1978). *Language development and language disorders.* New York: Wiley.

Bretherton, I., and Beeghly, M. (1982). Talking about internal states: The acquisition of an explicit theory of mind. *Developmental Psychology, 18,* 906–921.

Bretherton, I., McNew, S., Snyder, L., and Bates, E. (1983). Individual differences at 20 months: Analytic and holistic strategies of language acquisition. *Journal of Child Language, 10,* 293–320.

Brown, R. (1958). How shall a thing be called? *Psychological Review, 65,* 14–21.

Carey, S. (1982). Semantic development: The state of the art. In E. Wanner and L. Gleitman (Eds.). *Language acquisition: The state of the art.* New York: Cambridge.

Crystal, D. (1979). *Working with LARSP.* New York: Elsevier.

Crystal, D., Fletcher, P., and Garman, M. (1976). *The grammatical analysis of language disability.* New York: Elsevier.

Gallagher, T., and Darnton, B. (1978). Conversational aspects of language disordered children: Revision behaviors. *Journal of Speech and Hearing Research, 21,* 118–135.

Hall, W., and Nagy, W. (1981). Cultural differences in communication. *New York University Education Quarterly, 13,* 16–22.

Helmick, J., Watamori, T., and Palmer, J. (1976). Spouses' understanding of the communication disabilities of aphasic patients. *Journal of Speech and Hearing Disorders, 41,* 238–243.

Holland, A. (1976). Reply to Helmick et al. *Journal of Speech and Hearing Disorders, 41,* 438.

Holland, A., (1980). *CADL: Communicative abilities in daily living.* Baltimore: University Park Press.

Holland, A., (1982). Observing functional communication of aphasic adults. *Journal of Speech and Hearing Disorders, 47,* 50–56.

Holland, A., Miller, J., Reinmuth, O., et al. (1985). Rapid recovery from aphasia: A detailed language analysis. *Brain and Language, 24,* 156–173.

Johnson, D. (1974). The influence of social class and race on language test performance and spontaneous speech of preschool children. *Child Development, 45,* 517–521.

Kearns, K., and Simmons, N. (1983). A practical procedure for the grammatical analysis of aphasic language impairments: The LARSP. In Brookshire, R. (Ed.), *Clinical Aphasiology Conference Proceedings: 1983:* Minneapolis: BRK.

Kramer, C.A., James, S.L., and Saxman, J.H. (1979). A comparison of language samples elicited at home and in the clinic. *Journal of Speech and Hearing Disorders, 44,* 321–330.

Labov, W. (1976). Systematically misleading data from test questions. *The Urban Review, 9,* 146–169.

Lee, L. (1974). *Developmental sentence analysis.* Evanston, IL: Northwestern University Press.

Leonard, L., Schwartz, R., Morris, B., and Chapman, K. (1981). Factors influencing early lexical acquisition: Lexical orientation and phonological composition. *Child Development, 52,* 882–887.

Longhurst, T., and File, J. (1977). A comparision of developmental sentence scores from Head Start children collected in four conditions. *Language, Speech and Hearing Services in the Schools, 8,* 54–64.

MacWhinney, B. (1982). Basic syntactic processes. In S. Kuczaj (Ed.), *Language development: Syntax and semantics.* Hillsdale, NJ: Erlbaum.

MacWhinney, B., Bates, E., and Kliegl, R. (1984). Cue validity and sentence interpretation in English, German and Italian. *Journal of Verbal Learning and Verbal Behavior, 23,* 127–150.

Miller, J. (1981). *Assessing language production in children:* Baltimore: University Park Press.

Miller, J. and Chapman, R. (1983). *SALT: Systematic analysis of language transcripts, users' manual.* Madison: University of Wisconsin.

Nelson, K. (1982). Experimental gambits in the service of language acquisition theory. In S. Kuczaj, (Ed.) *Language development: Syntax and semantics.* Hillsdale, NJ: Erlbaum.

Newhoff, M., Tonkovich, J., Schwartz, S., and Burgess, E. (1982). Revision strategies in aphasia. In R. Brookshire (Ed.), *Clinical Aphasiology Conference Proceedings: 1982.* Minneapolis: BRK.

Olswang, L., and Carpenter, R. (1978). Elicitor effects on the language obtained from young language-impaired children. *Journal of Speech and Hearing Disorders, 43,* 76–88.

Penn, M.A.C. (1983). Syntactic and pragmatic aspects of aphasic language. Unpublished doctoral dissertation, University of the Witwatersrand, South Africa.

Quirk, R., Greenbaum, S., Leech, G., and Svartvik, J. (1972). *A grammar of contemporary English.* London: Longman.

Seymour, H., and Miller-Jones, D. (1981). Language and cognitive assessment of black children. In N. Lass (Ed.), *Speech and language: Advances in basic research and practice (Vol. 4).* New York: Academic Press.

Scott, C.M., and Taylor, A.E. (1978). A comparison of home and clinic gathered language samples. *Journal of Speech and Hearing Disorders, 43,* 482–495.

Snyder, L., Bates, E., and Bretherton, I. (1981). Content and context in early lexical development. *Journal of Child Language, 8,* 565–582.

Swindell, C., Pashek, G., and Holland, A. (1982). A questionnaire for surveying personal and communicative style. In R.H. Brookshire (Ed.), *Clinical Aphasiology Conference Proceedings: 1982.* Minneapolis: BRK.

Tyack, D., and Gottsleben, R. (1974). *Language sampling, analysis and training. A handbook for teachers and clinicians.* Palo Alto, CA: Consulting Psychologists Press.

Ylvisaker, M. (1983). *Infant communication questionnaire.* Unpublished manuscript.

Chapter 4

Cognitive Assessment of Nonwhite Children

Boris E. Bogatz,
Toshi Hisama,
John L. Manni,
and Reesa G. Wurtz

BACKGROUND

The significant overinclusion of minority children in the special education programs of this country has been well documented (Bogatz, 1976; Dunn, 1968; Jones, 1972; Lilly, 1970, 1971; Oakland, 1976). It is clear that Blacks, Hispanics, Asian-Americans, Native-Americans and other minority group students are being done a severe injustice by being diagnosed in highly disproportionate numbers as mildly handicapped because of assessment processes that would appear to be severely flawed. As a result of these questionable assessments, specialists in communication disorders may receive faulty information on the status of cognitive function, which undergirds all communicative behavior, normal as well as pathological. At the very heart of this situation lies the use of intelligence tests, which are culturally, racially, and linguistically biased in favor of the majority culture for which the tests were developed and on whose norms the tests have been standardized (*Larry P. v. Wilson Riles,* 1979).

The negative impact of being misdiagnosed and inappropriately placed in a special education program has been equally well documented (Dunn, 1968, 1973; Jones, 1972; Lilly, 1971). Hobbs (1974) enumerates the following effects of the classification and labeling that derive from special class placement.

1. Children who are categorized and labeled as different may be permanently stigmatized, rejected by adults and other children, and excluded from opportunities essential for their full and healthy development.
2. Children may be assigned to inferior educational programs for years, deprived of their liberty by being committed to an institution, or even sterilized on the basis of inadequate diagnostic procedures, with little or no consideration of due process.
3. Large numbers of minority group children — Chicanos, Puerto Ricans, Blacks, Appalachian whites — have been inaccurately classified as mentally retarded on the basis of inappropriate intelligence tests, placed in special classes or programs where stimulation and learning opportunities are inadequate, and stigmatized.

Futhermore, it is generally accepted that a "self-fulfilling prophecy" frequently develops and is greatly influenced by a presumed IQ score. A self-fulfilling prophecy is described as a situation in which a person

> prophesies an event and the expectation of the event then changes the behavior of the prophet in such a way as to make the prophesied event more likely. (Merton, 1948, p. 193).

A classic application of this notion has been described by Rosenthal and Jacobson (1966). These researchers showed that preconceived perceptions of a student's ability influenced the interaction between teacher and student resulting in significant differences in student performance. Teachers expected less and therefore taught less to youngsters who were assumed to have lower IQs than they did with youngsters who were thought to be more capable.

Recognition of these issues and the advent of Public Law 94–142 more recently has led segments of the special education community to attempt a variety of solutions. Some specific examples — such as pluralistic assessment and dynamic assessment (test-train-retest) procedures — are discussed later in this chapter. At present, federal law and regulations, as well as court interpretations, mandate that nondiscriminatory testing be assured to any youngster being considered for special education services of any type, including speech pathology and audiology services.

During the 1970s, the Regional Resource Center Network, through the Coordinating Office of Regional Resource Centers

(CORRC), spearheaded several nationwide efforts, which led to the establishment of guidelines for nondiscriminatory testing procedures (Bogatz, 1976, 1977; Oakland, 1976). Early on, there was difficulty in identifying relevant concerns because of the great disparity from state to state with respect to issues such as types of tests used, the ways test data were interpreted, and the required qualifications of test administrators.

The term "nondiscriminatory assessment" has created a good deal of controversy and discussion among psychologists and other professionals. There is often little consensus as to what the term means, and even less as to how it is achieved. Indeed, the phrase nondiscriminatory assessment may represent a contradiction of terms because all tests discriminate. Otherwise they would be useless. Those assessment instruments or assessment practices that discriminate unfairly on the basis of cultural background, race, or language, however, are in need of careful scrutiny. These tests and practices can be said to be *biased* either for or against a particular group, giving rise to the term "nonbiased assessment" as a more realistic way of referring to an assessment procedure that will not erroneously place minority group children into Special Education programs. It has since been suggested that some degree of bias is inherent in any interaction involving two or more human beings so that "least-biased" rather than "nonbiased" assessment might be still more appropriate terminology, reflecting a more realizable goal.

It should be noted that the terms "assessment," "evaluation," and "appraisal" are frequently used interchangeably. There is little consensus among professionals as to which term best describes the process of identifying and interpreting individual differences for determining valid diagnostic categories and appropriate educational planning. The term assessment as used in this chapter implies more than merely testing for the purpose of labeling or categorizing. Assessment is taken to mean a comprehensive process that incorporates all relevant aspects of behavior and environment and yields data upon which appropriate intervention strategies and educational programming are based.

The use of standardized intelligence tests with racially or culturally different children and the subsequent overrepresentation of these children in special education programs have been heatedly debated in scientific circles, as well as in courts and legislative bodies, throughout the United States. It has been clearly established through federal legislation and litigation that when IQ tests are used to assign children to educational programs, test bias cannot be evaluated solely on the basis of the instrument's psychometric properties. Social consequences, such as the highly disproportionate overinclusion of minority group youngsters in special education programs for the mildly handicapped, must also be considered. The role that the law and its interpretations have come to play sometimes arouses frustration, resistance, and even anger among professionals who perceive recent legal challenges as an assault on their professional competence and good intentions.

From a broader perspective, the proliferation of lawsuits and legislation with respect to special education can be viewed, at least in part, as a manifestation of the conflicts and tensions that characterized American society of the 1960s and 1970s. Significant segments of the society were attempting to focus public attention on a variety of social problems and needs. As a result, public education, as well as many other social institutions and agencies, came under attack.

In retrospect, it is clear that the many reforms that grew out of that era have resulted in an expansion of our consciousness and helped form a society that is far more aware of and considerably more sensitive and responsive to the needs of minority groups. In terms of the social science community, academicians and clinicians have had to evaluate the impact of their research and professional practices on minority group children. Because of the legal changes spawned during these turbulent years, psychologists and educators who wish to employ unbiased professional assessment practices with minority students must develop an awareness and understanding of the complex legal, ethical, and social parameters that have been shown to impact on the assessment of minority group youngsters.

LEGAL PERSPECTIVE

Before discussing court cases relevant to the use of IQ tests, we need to examine the relationship of the judiciary to public education. In 1954, the Supreme Court of the United States declared the public school practice of segregating children on the basis of race unconstitutional (*Brown v. Board of Education of Topeka,* 1954). Prior to this action, the judiciary had allowed educators broad powers with respect to the conduct of public education (Kuriloff, 1975). Legal scholars recognized this decision as a major change in the Court's stance and interpreted it as a victory for the civil rights movement. It also signaled a willingness on the part of the Supreme Court to enter the educational arena if school laws, regulations, or policies infringed upon the constitutional rights of children.

Since the Brown decision, civil rights advocates have turned with regularity to the courts for redress of discriminatory practices. The first case in which a court found tests to be discriminatory was *Hobson v. Hansen* (1967). The issue adjudicated in this case stemmed from the Washington, D.C., school system's practice of assigning students to educational tracks primarily on the basis of scores earned on standardized aptitude tests. As a result, a disproportionate number of black children were being assigned to the lower tracks. In this precedent-setting case, Judge V. Skelley Wright stated

> The evidence shows that the method by which track assignments are made depends essentially on standardized aptitude tests, which although given on a systematic basis, are completely inappropriate for use with a large segment of the student body. Because tests are standardized primarily on and are relevant to a white middle class group of students, they produce inaccurate and misleading test scores when given to lower class Negro students. . . . (p. 514)

Although the *Hobson v. Hansen* decision concerned group testing practices, it was not long before the use of individual IQ tests with racially or culturally different children was brought to the attention of the courts. The validity of the IQ test and the consequences of its use with racially or culturally different children were central issues, the resolution of which would have considerable bearing on assessment practices. In general, courts were asked to rule on the contention that IQ tests were biased, leading to significant overrepresentation of minority children in programs for the educable mentally retarded (EMR) and related social programs.

The first such case to be heard (*Diana v. California State Board of Education,* 1969) was filed as a class action suit on behalf of Mexican-American children who had been placed in EMR classes on the basis of standardized individually administered intelligence tests. Plaintiffs argued that children of Hispanic ethnic and linguistic backgrounds were overrepresented in EMR classes as the result of having been evaluated in English with tests which were culturally and linguistically biased. The suit was resolved through a consent decree stipulating that assessment procedures must take account of a child's native language and sociocultural background. Several thousand children in EMR classes were subsequently reevaluated with many being "decertified" and returned to regular classes. Another class action suit (*Guadalupe v. Tempe Elementary School District,* 1971) in Arizona on behalf of Mexican-American and Yaqui Indian children had similar results.

The overrepresentation of Black children in EMR classes as a result of their performance on individually administered intelligence tests was the focus of the *Stewart v. Phillips* (1970) suit. Plaintiffs contended that Black children who had been inappropriately classified as educable mentally retarded and placed in special education programs had suffered irreparable damage. Consequently, monetary compensation was sought, but the case was settled out of court without the awarding of damages.

One of the most recent cases (*Larry P. v. Wilson Riles,* 1979) is also one that promises to have significant impact on assessment practices. Known as "Larry P.," this suit was originally filed in 1971 on behalf of six Black children in California who were classified as mentally retarded by the San Francisco Unified School District. Eight years later, on October 16, 1979, Federal District Court Judge Robert R. Peckham handed down his decision in favor of the plaintiffs' assertion that standardized IQ tests (1) are racially and culturally biased, therefore discriminating against Black children, and (2) have not been validated for the purpose of educational placement.

When the suit was filed, Blacks constituted 28.5 percent of the San Francisco school system and 66 percent of the EMR population. It was the opinion of the court that Black children were grossly overrepresented in EMR classes because individually administered tests of intelligence that are racially and culturally biased against minority children had been used. The court further found that intelligence tests had not been validated for the purpose of placement decisions involving Black children and that their impact upon Black children was clearly discriminatory. The State of California was enjoined from further use of such tests without specific approval by the court. This decision has recently been upheld by the United States Court of Appeals, Ninth Circuit (1984).

The PASE case (*Parents in Action on Special Education v. Joseph P. Hannon, et al.,* 1980) once again raised the issue of overrepresentation of Black children in EMR classes. Rather than relying on the arguments put forth in Larry P., however, plaintiffs questioned the use of IQ tests with Black students on the basis of the test's content validity. After examining items in the Wechsler Intelligence Scale, the court determined that such tests were not biased. The nature of the Judge's approach has been questioned (Manni, Winikur, and Keller, 1984). Futhermore, the recent failure to overturn Larry P. on appeal suggests that the arguments presented by the plaintiffs and the decision rendered by Judge Peckham set a more appropriate path for administrators and clinicians.

The federal government has also attempted to address the issue of overrepresentation of minority students in EMR classes. Both the Rehabilitation Act of 1973 and the Education of All Handicapped Children Act of 1975 (PL 94–142) attempted to set standards for evaluation materials and procedures. Although both sets of standards are similar, PL 94–142 will be cited because educators are most familiar with its regulations. Congress clearly intended to address the issue of bias with respect to the evaluation of minority children by including this statement in the statute (U.S.C. 141 2 [5] [c]):

> Procedures to assure that testing and evaluation materials and procedures utilized for the purposes of evaluation and placement of handicapped children will be selected and administered so as not to be racially or culturally discriminatory. Such materials or procedures shall be provided and administered in the child's native language or mode of communication unless it clearly is not feasible to do so and no single procedure shall be the sole criterion for determining an appropriate educational program for a child (Education of All Handicapped Children Act, 1975).

Two years later regulations were published for PL 94–142 that clearly set forth "Protection in Evaluation Procedures" (Federal Register, 1977). Essentially the regulations require that, at a minimum, state and local education agencies shall ensure that tests and other evaluation materials

1. Are provided and administered in the child's native language or other mode of communication, unless it is clearly not feasible to do so;
2. Have been validated for the specific purpose for which they are used;
3. Are administered by trained personnel in conformance with the instructions provided by their producer;
4. Tests and other evaluation materials include those tailored to assess specific areas of educational need and not merely those that are designed to provide a single general intelligence quotient;
5. Tests are selected and administered so as best to ensure that when a test is administered to a child with impaired sensory, manual, or speaking skills, the test results accurately reflect the child's aptitude or achievement level or whatever other factors the test purports to measure, rather than reflecting the child's impaired sensory, manual, or speaking skills (except where those skills are the factors that the test purports to measure);
6. No single procedure is used as the sole criterion for determining an appropriate educational program for a child;
7. The evaluation is made by a multidisciplinary team or group of

persons, including at least one teacher or other specialist with a knowledge in the area of suspected disability;
8. The child is assessed in all areas related to the suspected disability, including, where appropriate, health, vision, hearing, social and emotional status, general intelligence, academic performance, communicative status, and motor abilities.

THE QUESTION OF BIAS

The question of whether IQ tests are biased against certain sociocultural groups has long been debated from a psychometric perspective. For a thorough review of this issue, the reader is referred to works by Blanton (1975), Brody and Brody (1976), Gould (1981), Kamin (1974), and Manni and colleagues (1984), which recapitulate the arguments in detail. Suffice it to say here that there has always existed a school of thought that attributes the mean differences found between racially and culturally diverse groups to genetic endowment. Other groups have argued against this position, suggesting that performance on IQ tests is heavily influenced by environmental forces. The authors of this chapter adhere to the position that intelligence is multifaceted and results from a complex interaction of genetic endowment and environmental factors. Substantial support of this position has been offered by theoreticians and researchers such as Brody and Brody (1976), Gould (1981), and Scarr (1981). Hence, the frequently cited finding that the mean performance of white children is approximately 15 points higher than the mean performance of Black children on intelligence tests (Brody and Brody, 1976; Kaufman and Dappelt, 1976; Shuey, 1966) does not, in the authors' opinion, reflect innate, genetic differences. Rather, it is seen as an artifact of an assessment procedure that measures differences in environmental influences, cultural heritage, and language, not as a deficiency in cognitive ability of the children.

With respect to the use of IQ tests for minority children, the central question is one of validity. Messick (1980) suggests that an evaluation of a test's validity must include an examination of the adequacy of the instrument and appraisal of its social consequences. The authors do not take exception to the psychometric adequacy of instruments such as the Wechsler Intelligence Scale for Children – Revised (WISC-R). However, the meaning ascribed to the scores derived from such tests and the social consequences of their use are questionable. In the past, IQ scores have been used to evaluate intellectual status regardless of the student's social or cultural background. In addition, the tests have often been the major vehicle by which minority children were assigned to EMR classes. It has been argued successfully in the courts that although minority children who perform poorly on intelligence tests may indeed lack the skills IQ tests measure, it cannot be assumed that their performance is the result of limited intellectual ability. As Judge Peckham put it aptly:

> While many think of the IQ as an objective measure of innate, fixed intelligence, the testimony of the experts overwhelmingly demonstrated that this conception of IQ is erroneous. Defendants' expert witnesses, even those closely affiliated with the companies that devise and distribute the standardized intelligence tests, agreed, with one exception, that we cannot truly define, much less measure, intelligence. We can measure certain skills but not native intelligence. Professor Robert Thorndike of Columbia, defendants' first expert witness, confirmed that the modern consensus represents a change from that held in the early years of the testing movement: "Everybody would acknowledge we would have no conceivable way of directly measuring native ability." Dr. Leo Munday, Vice President and General Manager, Test Department, Houghton Mifflin Co., publishers of the Stanford-Binet, similarly concluded that, "It is safe to say that . . . no one in aptitude testing today believes that intelligence tests measure innate capacity. *IQ tests, like other ability tests, essentially measure achievement skills covered by the examinations."* (pp. 37–38) (italics added)

Problems related to the cognitive assessment of Asian American children are similarly complex. First, there is a lack of awareness regarding the extent of diversity within the Asian American group itself. Second, the complexity of Asian languages is such that the bilingual approach applicable to Indo-European languages may not be appropriate. Third, the impact of minority group status on Asian American handicapped children may be particularly severe because of the intense identity crisis that often develops in these youngsters.

It is a commonly held misconception that Asian Americans constitute a single group with common characteristics. A stereotypic notion is that they all look alike, and therefore they all think, behave, and act alike. In the United States, there are more than half a million Americans of Japanese descent, and the number of the Chinese-Americans far exceeds that. In addition, there are Koreans, Filipinos, Indonesians, Thais, Indians, Cambodians, Pakistanis, Burmese, Vietnamese, Micronesians, and other peoples, each with cultural and linguistic backgrounds so diverse that it is ludicrous to generalize about them under one label, be it Asian American or any other. Their languages, child-rearing patterns, attitudes toward education, achievement motivation, and other cultural characteristics are as much different as those of Blacks in the United States and Blacks in Zaire, for instance.

Assuming that there is no difference in genetic endowment between Anglo-Americans and Orientals, studies tend to emphasize the effect of environmental factors, particularly bilingualism, on the assessment of cognitive development. Second-generation Japanese born in the United States (Nisei) were typically brought up speaking Japanese, and it was not unusual for Nisei children to learn English for the first time when they attended elementary school. The linguistic and educational environment of Nisei children was, therefore, very similar to that of Hispanics, particularly Mexican-Americans, in today's society.

We must also be aware that there is a great deal of diversity even within one ethnic group. Many first generation Japanese-Americans (Issei), for example, totally retained the culture from the old country. Nisei (second generation Japanese-Americans) are situated between the Issei and the Sansei (third generation) in terms of their cultural assimilation, and Yonsei (fourth generation) are totally "American" and, unlike the Issei, Nisei, and Sansei, speak only English.

This "minority-within-a-minority" status of ethnic groups among the Asian American community and Native American groups is often unrecognized by the public (Wagner, 1977). Referring to these groups as the "hyphenated Americans," Sata (1977) emphasized the diversity that exists between and among groups. It has been estimated that, among the Native American population, there exist some 400 different tribal and linguistic heritages. Obviously, if we are concerned with cultural, linguistic, and ethnic parity in the assessment of cognitive function, we cannot refer to the "Native American" except in a very general sense.

This diversity and identity problem bears directly on cognitive assessment. Evidence strongly indicates that testing a child in a nondominant language can seriously depress the score achieved. Many practical problems arise, however, in trying to conduct an assessment in each of the many languages that may be dominant among the Asian American and Native American communities. Consider, for example, the influx of immigrants from countries such as Vietnam and Laos and the fact that, as recently as 1980, the Illinois Registry of Bilingual Examiners (Crowner, 1980) listed only two Vietnamese and one Laotian as qualified examiners in these languages.

Test items, or context, can be significantly biased against Asian American and Native American children. An item on the WISC-R asks, for example, what the child should do if he or she finds that the grocery store does not have bread when the child is sent on an errand. A standard two point answer is that the child should go to another grocery store even though it often happens that a reservation has only one grocery store.

Examiners and the values they hold can negatively influence the assessment process. Respect for authority, filial piety, and "saving face" are common threads among Chinese and Japanese children (Chinn, 1983), and similar reaction patterns are noted among other Asian American children. These characteristics are often mistaken by American teachers and assessors for passivity, disinterest, negativism, laziness, and lack of intellectual aptitude.

A variety of studies have documented the impact of cultural and linguistic differences of Asian American children. Yoshioka (1929) reported that the average score of the Asian American children was far below the average score of American children on the National Intelligence Test. Yoshioka attributed the lower score of the Japanese children in California to their bilingual environment at home. Smith (1957), in an extensive study of preschool children of "non-American" ancestry in Hawaii, reached the same conclusion. She found that when children were brought up in an environment in which "Pidgin English" was the main means of communication, cognitive functioning as reflected on intelligence tests appeared much lower than that of children on the mainland. Obviously, a child's performance on a standardized test may be negatively affected by language differences.

Portenier (1945) studied the abilities and intellect of Japanese-American high school seniors who were interned in relocation camps during World War II.* Japanese-American students were found to have a median IQ of 97.61 on the Henmon-Nelson Test, a score inferior to that of white counterparts. Anxiety, depression, anger, feelings of helplessness, and hopelessness were reported as common factors among the Japanese in relocation camps and no doubt contributed to the low scores.

An earlier study (Sandiford and Kerr, 1926) employed the Pintner-Patterson Scale of Performance Test, which is less culturally influenced. The results yielded a median IQ of 115.4 for Japanese boys and a median IQ of 112.8 for Japanese girls with similar results reported for a Chinese group. Although the results pointed to the ef-

---

*Japanese-Americans on the West Coast were regarded as potential enemies during World War II and were confined to relocation camps.

fectiveness of using a performance scale instead of a verbal scale, the authors attributed the "surprising" finding to the selective migration theory (i.e., a smart and aggressive group migrated to the United States and Canada, whereas a more docile and unambitious group stayed in the home country.

Studies with Chinese-Americans consistently report findings that document the negative effects of bilingualism on the assessment of cognitive function. Smith and Kasdon (1961), for example, studied 151 four and five year old Japanese-American and Filipino-American children, clearly showing that despite a dramatic increase in the use of English words, Asian American children were one half to 1 full year behind the norm in their language age performance on standardized tests. Pidgin English, the authors reported, still greatly influenced language performance of children of the three ethnic groups on tests written in standard English.

In a recent cross-cultural study, Lynn (1982) compared the IQ of children in Japan and the United States and reported that the mean IQ in Japan is higher than in the United States by approximately one third to two thirds of a standard deviation. Results indicated an average performance IQ of 111 for the Japanese children compared with an average IQ of 100 for American children. Lynn also points out that whereas 2 percent of American and European populations have IQs over 130, 10 percent of Japanese are above this level. Among the population as a whole, 77 percent of Japanese have a higher IQ than the average American or European, although the results of this study have been challenged (Flynn, 1983; Vining, 1983).

A variety of studies (Dennis, 1942; Havighurst, Gunther, and Pratt, 1946; Rohrer, 1942; Wilson, 1973) clearly indicate that Native American children possess average to above average cognitive functioning when this ability is measured by the Draw-a-Man Test and other performance oriented instruments. Results are dramatically different, however, when the assessment requires language responses. A recent study (Naglieri and Yazzie, 1983) reported that the results of administering the WISC-R and the Wechsler Primary and Pre-School Scale of Intelligence (WPPSI) to Native American children clearly indicated a lag in verbal intelligence development, whereas performance intelligence was within the normal range. Navajo children, for example, achieved a mean verbal IQ of 74.9 and an average performance IQ of 103.8 on the WISC-R. Clearly, these results demonstrate that these children score in the average to superior range when tested with instruments that are appropriate to their cultural and linguistic experiences.

ASSESSMENT ALTERNATIVES

Intelligence is a scientific construct. The relationship between presently constituted IQ tests and intelligence continues to be disputed. Brody and Brody (1976) contend that IQ scores "are only tenuously related to the construct they allegedly measure and it requires a rather elaborate inference to assert that they are measures of the construct" (p. 200). Accordingly, intelligence test scores should not be interpreted as valid indicators of innate capacity, and they do not necessarily remain fixed throughout life (Reschly, 1979). IQ tests are considered moderately good predictors of performance on achievement tests (Reschly, 1980). With this in mind, IQ tests can be thought of as assessing the extent to which any child has acquired the information necessary for success in our schools. Children who perform poorly on intelligence tests are not likely to perform well in school. It must not be assumed, however, that their poor performance is the result of limited intellectual capacity. IQ tests can be used validly with minority group children if the results are used to ascertain what a child has and has not learned. IQ scores cannot validly be used to define the limits of a racially or culturally different child's potential for learning.

As has been suggested earlier, many studies have demonstrated that children from certain sociocultural and socioeconomic groups perform significantly below established middle class norms. In general, the results of these studies suggest that intelligence tests, as they are currently used, do not accurately reflect the qualitative and quantitative differences they purport to measure (Feuerstein and Rand, 1977; Mercer, 1975; Williams, 1974). Test abuse has also been of particular concern, specifically in the "over-evaluation of global IQs, equation of test scores with genetic potential and interpretation of low IQs as a call to passive placement rather than active intervention" (Kaufman, 1979, p. 2).

Owing to the limitations of standardized intelligence tests, concerned educators are aggressively seeking new ways of assessing a child's cognitive functioning. Responses can be categorized as (1) modification of existing instruments, (2) the development of new assessment procedures, or (3) designing assessment processes that encompass extant tests in ways that ensure nonbiased application.

System of Multicultural Pluralistic Assessment (SOMPA)

One example of a modification made in testing procedures occurs in the use of the WISC-R (Wechsler, 1974) when employed as a part of the System of Multicultural Pluralistic Assessment (SOMPA) (Mercer and Lewis, 1977). Mercer acknowledges that standardized tets are culturally biased in favor of the Anglo-American majority culture, but includes the WISC-R in the SOMPA package with some modifications in interpretation. In addition, other measures included in the SOMPA, such as the Adaptive Behavior Inventory for Children (ABIC), ensure that the IQ test will not be given in isolation. This practice is also in compliance with Public Law 94–142 regulations that specify multifactored, unbiased assessment.

The SOMPA is a system of tests developed to assess children from culturally different backgrounds. The evaluation process is systematic in that three different models of assessment are used, with many of the specific measures included already familiar to psychologists and educators. Children are examined comprehensively with tests that operate from a Medical Model perspective, a Social System perspective, and Pluralistic perspective, each having its own definitions, assumptions, characteristics, measurement properties, and ethical code.

As stated, the WISC-R is included in the Social System and Pluralistic models. Under the Social System model, the WISC-R IQ score is interpreted as the School Functioning Level (SFL), measuring behavior appropriate for success in the school. Based on the high IQ correlation to academic achievement (.5 to .7), Mercer suggests that standardized IQ scores should be "interpreted as a prediction of how well a particular child is likely to do in the academic role in the public schools" (1979, p. 149). In the Pluralistic Model, the WISC-R is applied in a way that compares a child only with others from similar sociocultural environments through the use of multiple norms. Scores obtained here are referred to as the Estimated Learning Potential (ELP).

The use of multiple norms is the most controversial aspect of the SOMPA. The ELP score cannot be determined without administration of the Sociocultural Scales to the parent, which produces a score that is used to "correct" the WISC-R score through means of regression equations. A new score, the Estimated Learning Potential, is determined according to ethnic group (Black, white, Hispanic). The ELP indicates how a child's skills compare with those of other youngsters of the same age and sociocultural background. According to Mercer (1979), the ELP will more closely approximate a child's true learning potential because sociocultural effects have been taken into account.

The ELP has been criticized for several of its characteristics. The development or modification of IQ norms to be used with the culturally disadvantaged has, generally, been considered a less than adequate answer to the inappropriateness of tests for this group. According to Feuerstein (1979), scores obtained from "local norms" function to rank a child in relation to other members of his own group. However, the development of new norms implies that these individuals are (inherently) inferior in comparison to the majority group because the standardized norms were considered inappropriate. Feuerstein further states that

> The results may therefore serve to deepen the negative stereotype in regard to the disadvantaged groups. The danger inherent in the development of special norms is that culturally disadvantaged individuals' functioning is eventually interpreted as substantiating the viewpoint that immutable genetic and constitutional factors determine his low level of functioning, as in the stable deficit models of Shuey (1966) and Jenson (1969). (p. 40)

The ELP has also been criticized for lack of empirical evidence establishing its validity. According to Oakland (1979, 1980) the ELP does not relate as highly as the IQ score to measure of academic achievement (.40 and .60, respectively). Therefore, the value and usage of the ELP score is questionable.

In a study by Wurtz (1981) of 31 Black and 32 white EMR children, the ELP and SFL were employed as predictor variables with performance on a learning task as the criterion. Although the ELP did not predict performance better than the SFL, the ELP score did tend to be more sensitive in the differential diagnosis of both Black and white children. That is, the ELP score was determined to be more appropriate in the "decertification" of children previously diagnosed as retarded.

The SOMPA, therefore, may be considered a middle-of-the-road approach to solving the problem of appropriate use of standardized tests. The battery itself ensures that areas other than "intelligence" will be measured and that educational intervention will be based upon additional measures as well. Furthermore, the ELP, which is not another IQ score, aids in the appropriate assessment of the child because sociocultural factors are used for its interpretation.

Dynamic Assessment (Learning Potential Assessment)

Another modification of current assessment practices occurs in procedures of test administration rather than in the content of the tests. This approach, often referred to as Dynamic Assessment, focuses upon the process of intellectual functioning with emphasis on how it may be improved (Feuerstein, 1979).

Dynamic assessment is understood best through a comparison with more traditional measures. First, a dynamic approach attempts to assess the extent to which a child's level of cognitive functioning can be modified by an investment of teaching effort. Therefore, the assessment paradigm follows a test-teach-test model in contrast to conventional, norm-referenced tests of cognitive functioning, which measure skills that exist at the time of testing and allow for no intervention as a part of the procedure. Second, the teaching component of the dynamic assessment strategy encourages the child to apply problem-solving strategies learned during the assessment to progressively more difficult items. Traditional testing instruments do not usually include items that are sensitive to learning, owing to the tendency of those items to adversely affect reliability of measures.

There are other differences between conventional evaluation practice and "learning potential assessment" procedures, as referred to by Budoff (1972) and Feuerstein (1979). The examiner-examinee relationship, usually one in which interaction is limited to neutral administration of standardized instructions, becomes one of teacher-pupil interaction. That is, both examiner and child are involved in a mutual goal — the accomplishment of the goal. Learning potential assessment, with its process orientation, provides opportunities to examine the child's approach to the task as well as the quality of response. Of interest also is the extent to which intervention by the examiner is needed to promote appropriate responding (i.e., cueing, modeling, task analysis). The results of the interaction are seen as useful for purposes of remediation and educational intervention.

Inadequate performance on IQ tests is, according to Feuerstein, reflected by the "underdeveloped, poorly developed, arrested and/or impaired" cognitive functions often characteristic of the culturally disadvantaged (1979, p. 57). Feuerstein believes that this "state of impairment" is caused by the lack of opportunity for the child to engage in what he refers to as "mediated learning experiences" (p. 70). Mediated learning occurs during periods of adult-child interaction when the adult helps the child attend to or manipulate objects. That is, the adult interprets the environment to the child, and encourages "appropriate learning sets and habits" (p. 71). Therefore, cognitive deficiencies do not necessarily occur because of neurological impairment or poor genetic endowment but as a result of the absence of or poor quality of adult-child interaction, affecting the child's appropriate response to his environment. Thus, the training portion of the procedure is designed to mediate the learning experiences for the child.

Dynamic assessment yields an index of cognitive modifiability.

The initial testing in the test-teach-test model attempts to obtain a baseline performance, which is compared to performance during training and retesting. Feuerstein contends that the assessment of intelligence requires evaluation of skills at three levels of information processing. Learning potential is ultimately evaluated by measuring the extent to which a child can grasp a new principle, learning set, or skill, according to the task. The capacity of the child for modifiability and the amount of teaching effort required to bring about change is assessed by measuring the child's ability to comprehend and then apply the new skills to new tasks.

The dynamic assessment approach offers great potential as an alternative to traditional assessment procedures, which have been shown to impact so negatively on minority group youngsters. When used with an educable mentally retarded (EMR) population, it has been demonstrated to be sensitive to those subjects who are educationally or experientially retarded rather than comprehensively retarded (Budoff and Corman, 1976; Wurtz, 1981). The following case study exemplifies the benefits of the dynamic assessment approach. The subject was one of 31 Black and 32 white children participating in a study utilizing the learning potential assessment strategy.

The subject was a Black youngster named James, aged 10 years 7 months, who attended an EMR class in a large urban school district. James's IQ scores, according to the WISC-R, were 69 on all three scores, Verbal, Performance, and Full Scale. He had been classified as retarded while in the second grade.

According to the Sociocultural Scales (SC) of the SOMPA, James was from a single-parent family that was dependent on public assistance. When the SC scales were used to obtain the Estimated Learning Potential, James's scores were found to be Verbal score, 84; Performance score, 82; Full Scale score, 82.

The learning potential assessment strategy was also employed using the Raven Progressive Matrices as a learning task. This was done to ascertain the degree to which James would benefit from instruction. The pretest found James to be functioning at the 10th percentile for his age group. This was followed by a 45-minute session of training on materials that were similar to the nonverbal problems of the Raven test. At this time the examiner also interacted with James and observed the degree of interaction necessary for James to respond appropriately.

Results of the pretest, which occurred one week later, found James to be performing at the 90th percentile for his age level, indicating that he had the potential for learning at a rate appropriate for his chronological age. Furthermore, his performance raised questions about his classification as educable mentally retarded. To what extent, for example, was his academic performance the result of cultural, ethnic, language, or experiential diversity rather than basic intelligence? Clearly, the Estimated Learning Potential score used in conjunction with the learning potential strategy confirmed that this youngster's potential was not accurately represented by the more conventional assessment techniques.

THE PROCESS OF NONBIASED ASSESSMENT

It must also be recognized that a nonbiased assessment process, which meets all of the legal and regulatory criteria, may be rendered ineffective or negated by administrative fiat. Tucker (1976) states that

> assessment techniques *per se* are not always responsible for discrimination. It is possible to accumulate sufficient information on a child to enable assessment specialists to provide a relatively unbiased decision. But if placement decisions are made by choosing to ignore professional judgment in favor of formulas, cut-off scores, or other traditional recipes for categorization that ignore cultural differences, then the data become tools used for a biased decision. (p. 44)

Tucker goes on to characterize a nonbiased assessment process as one that

(1) is ongoing
(2) results from a team effort
(3) involves the child's parents as active participants
(4) investigates all relevant data sources such as observations, historical data,* language dominance, educational achievement, sensorimotor development, adaptive behavior, medical or developmental history, personality, and intellectual development.

These data sources have been combined into an assessment that is first and foremost comprehensive (Fig. 4–1). Further, it relegates intellectual testing to the last step in the assessment process for determining a youngster's eligibility for special class placement (Tucker, 1976, p. 46).

Each data source is evaluated and provides input on which an appropriate decision is reached for that youngster. Only after determining that the data do support further investigation is the next step in the evaluation process implemented. A "no" response to any

---

*Tucker's original term was "other data available."

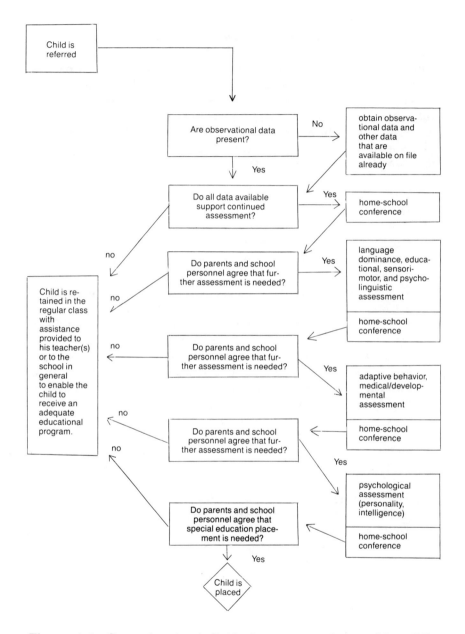

Figure 4–1. Comprehensive individual assessment for possible mildly handicapping conditions. From Tucker, J. A. (1976). Operationalizing the diagnostic-intervention process. In *With bias toward none: A national survey of assessment programs and procedures.* Lexington: University of Kentucky. Reprinted with permission.

decision point requires that the youngster be retained in (or returned to) the regular class, but with appropriate remedial assistance or other regular education alternatives provided as indicated. Intellectual testing, the final step, serves in a very real sense to corroborate all of the preceding assessment data rather than as an entity in and of itself. The IQ score, rather than establishing a self-fulfilling prophecy, would not even be known until all of the other assessment data have clearly indicated a need for special education placement. The nine assessment categories in Tucker's model are described as follows (pp. 47–51):

1. *Observational Data.* Before a child is considered for special education intervention, adequate information should be obtained from teachers and other educators who worked directly with and know the child. Such data should be required as support for the need for the referral. It is, in a sense, the child's first line of defense. Without such data in sufficient quantity, decision makers may act on the emotionally inspired request of a single person who wants a child moved [or removed]. Many times when sufficient observational data accompany the initial consideration for special education intervention it is a relatively simple matter to prescribe immediate intervention that does not require further assessment or [consideration for] special placement. The objective of gathering observational data is to obtain an indication of deviance or lack thereof from standards of normal children within the same educational environment.

2. *Other Data Available (Historical).* Observational data can be misleading if they represent a temporary situation in the child's life. By inspecting the child's cumulative records and other available data without additional testing, decision makers can ascertain if there are any other indications from the child's history that would account for the referred behavior. For example, if a child has been absent from school for more than he or she has been present, certain current behaviors could be explained easily in terms of that past history. Data from medical examinations or hearing and vision screening may be on record. Furthermore, if such information is not available, this suggests a need to request it from schools previously attended, from parents, or from other sources. The objective of checking available data is to locate corroborating or disconfirming evidence of the deviance observed.

3. *Language Dominance Data.* Determining a child's language dominance and degree to which it is compatible with the language used in the school can be critical in determining the de-

gree to which a child may or may not be exhibiting symptoms of a possible handicapping condition. Information on language dominance is needed primarily to avoid the misdiagnosis (and subsequent misplacement) of non-native English speaking pupils and to identify language deficiencies that need attention. The objective of ascertaining language dominance is to determine the language appropriate for further assessment and to determine the effects that language (or the lack thereof) may have on other data collected.

4. *Educational Assessment Data.* Under the available data section, general information about a child's academic progress was obtained. This information, however, may be an inaccurate reflection of the child's level of educational achievement or may be discrepant with the observational data reported with the referral. An in-depth, individually administered educational assessment often is necessary. The objectives of gathering additional educational data are to determine under more controlled conditions the child's functional educational abilities in subject matter areas and to determine if a discrepancy exists between a child's previously reported achievement and the level at which he or she is able to perform under more controlled conditions. The purpose here should be to provide a base for building an academically oriented intervention program.

5. *Sensorimotor Data.* The rationale is that sensorimotor difficulties are associated with learning handicaps and can be remedied, allowing for an increase in learning. The objective of gathering data from sensorimotor assessment is to establish support, or the lack thereof, for considering placement in a setting for the learning disabled. The data also may be useful for educational programming.

6. *Adaptive Behavior Data.* It is important to know the degree to which behavior observed in the learning environment is generalized to other environments — the playground, the home, the neighborhood, and the community. Many children who do not function in the normal range in the traditional learning environment are quite capable of normal functioning in nonacademic settings. Adaptive behavior measures permit us to ascertain if a child's general adaptive skills are similar to those of other children of the same age and enable the child to function effectively within his or her cultural or environmental setting. The primary consideration is in the degree to which the referred child's out-of-school behaviors are similar to his or her in-school behaviors.

7. *Medical or Developmental Data.* A child may show symptoms that appear to the casual observer as evidence of handicapping condi-

tions deserving special education intervention when in fact the child is suffering from a medical problem that can be remedied by medical intervention. It is important to know the medical and developmental history of a child when making decisions about educational programs that may affect him or her in unknown ways. The objective of gathering medical or developmental data is to provide assurance that difficulties observed are not medical in origin and to provide data that will serve as a basis for a referral for appropriate treatment.

8. *Personality Assessment Data.* Complex emotional and personality variables may interact in many ways to cause the child's referred behavior. It is quite helpful to have valid data regarding these variables. There may be nothing "handicapped" about the child, and his or her problem might be corrected by intervention strategies available through the regular school program (i.e., the school counselor). On the other hand, some form of psychosis and severe neurosis may be present and diagnosed, so appropriate special education intervention can be provided. It is especially important to get the child's own viewpoint of what is going on and how he or she perceives it by interviewing the child directly. Many times decisions are made which move children from place to place and no one ever asks the child what he or she thinks. The objective is to determine the degree of emotional involvement in the observed deviant behaviors and to determine the degree of abnormality, if any, present.

9. *Intellectual Assessment Data.* Tests of academic aptitudes are valuable tools which can provide objective, quantifiable, and predictive data. If one accepts that the basic role of school is to foster academic development, these tests provide the best predictors of success. It is when tests are used to classify pupils into ability levels for special education classes for the mentally retarded that problems arise. The objective of intellectual assessment is to provide accurate data to estimate the level of the child's intellectual functioning. The question to answer is, "what evidence exists in the data from all other sources to substantiate the findings of the intellectual assessment." If the answer is "little or none," it would be unthinkable to place any reliance on an IQ score regardless of how well the test was administered in accordance with strict standardized testing procedures. Let the weight of available data speak for itself, and never give added weight to the IQ test simply because it provides a score.

More recently, a comprehensive procedure for the nonbiased assessment of minority group youngsters was developed by the Washington, DC, public schools (Bogatz, 1981). The result of this significant effort was a comprehensive assessment manual containing a process which, if adhered to, would greatly reduce, if not eliminate, the occurrence of biased placement decisions. The process requires that a variety of regular education alternatives and interventions be attempted before a youngster can be referred for a more thorough assessment.

Specific nonbiased assessment questionnaires and checklists are built in at decision points that are particularly sensitive to the possibility of biased decisions. The process incorporates the multidimensional assessment data sources as described by Tucker (1976) and ensures that all relevant "data sources" are included at appropriate points in the assessment process.

Underlying the development of this process is the understanding that educational assessment is for the purpose of identifying the unique learning needs of individual students, thereby providing the basis for the development of successful educational interventions. The function of assessment, then, is to provide relevant decision makers with appropriate information for educational programming and planning, including placement in necessary related services such as speech-language therapy. Relevant decision makers in this scheme are referred to as an Interdisciplinary Team, composed of those individuals who (1) provide evaluative data necessary for the formulation of an Individual Educational Program (IEP) and (2) are responsible for its implementation. The importance of parent (and when possible student) participation in all aspects of the assessment process is recognized.

Components of the assessment are by necessity to be administered by skilled and knowledgeable examiners, using instruments and procedures that evaluate significant factors related to the learning process. Assessment, interpretation of assessment results, educational placement, and intervention planning are the responsibility, therefore, of an interdisciplinary team of persons who are knowledgeable about the student and about educational options and related services available. This is not to say that a given team will have the same composition throughout the process. Indeed, the team composition will no doubt be modified frequently as determined by the unique and changing needs of the student being assessed.

Assurance of continuing least restrictive and appropriate instructional interventions requires ongoing assessment of the individual's current levels of functioning and progress being made in accordance with the Individual Educational Program. Ongoing reassessment is therefore a prominent feature of this process.

A comprehensive assessment determines an individual student's current levels of functioning through the use of multiple assessment measures, thereby prohibiting any single assessment instrument or procedure from constituting the sole criterion on which an educational decision is made. Assessment instruments and techniques are selected within the context of specific assessment goals and with knowledge of the individual and his or her larger environment.

The assessment process is limited to the least restrictive assessment phase necessary and sufficient for the development of an optimal individual educational program. Assessment activities are discontinued at the earliest point within each phase on the assessment continuum at which the team agrees that sufficient information for planning has been obtained. This assessment process is characterized by a commitment to building on a child's strengths and capitalizing on the unique combination of each child's individual characteristics as well as his family, cultural, ethnic, and linguistic orientation.

The goal is an educational program that is designed to maximize each child's unique set of characteristics and abilities. The function of assessment, then, is to provide accurate information for educational programming and planning through an interdisciplinary team decision-making process. But what if members of the decision-making team hold different beliefs and assumptions about education and the learning process? Clearly one problem related to non-discriminatory assessment is the fact that each professional comes to the assessment with preconceived biases and perspectives about assessment, the educational process, and, indeed, children.

A statement of assumption is not necessarily a statement of fact. An assumption is a statement that is temporarily accepted as "true" until proved false. Assumptions provide the working foundation of "self-evident" or "accepted" truth until such time as the research provides a firmer empirical basis on which to rest decisions. The following policy statements and assumptions further describe the philosophical base on which this nonbiased assessment process was developed. Recognition of these statements further assures a common perspective.

POLICY STATEMENTS

1. That naturally occurring student characteristics such as race, sex, physical appearance, handicapping condition, native language, and other characteristics such as socioeconomic status, religion, or parental power shall not affect assessment decisions.

2. Tests and evaluation materials shall be selected and administered only by, or under the supervision of, persons who meet all applicable certification or license requirements. Evaluation results and interpretation shall be accepted only from those professionals whose training certifies skill in the use of the instruments from which data are derived.

3. Tests and evaluation materials shall be selected, administered, and interpreted in accordance with the purposes and instructions provided by the producer or author of such test materials. Evaluation instruments shall have demonstrated validity for the purpose for which they are used.

4. Educational assessments shall be derived from a preestablished list of instruments whose standardization procedures and reliability and validity coefficients are acceptable.

5. Assessment instruments shall be chosen and results interpreted on the basis of the specific decisions to be made. Norm and criterion referenced tests shall be used in the assessment of skill development and may be used as a part of the data collection.

6. Performance shall be reported in terms of age, grade, developmental, or maturational equivalents. Since IQs cannot be used as the sole criterion for educational programming, IQs without interpretation shall not be included in reports. Tests and evaluation materials shall include those tailored to assess specific areas of educational need and performance or ability, not merely those that are designed to provide a single general intelligence quotient.

7. Tests shall be administered in the primary language of the child by an examiner familiar with the language. Results shall be interpreted to and discussed with parents in their primary language.

8. Performance dimensions to be sampled routinely shall include cognition, language development, perception, motor development, and social and emotional adaptivity.

9. Tests and evaluation materials that are used to determine the aptitude or achievement of students with impaired sensory, manual, or speaking skills shall be designed for and be effective in determining actual sensory, manual, or speaking skills.

10. Written reports generated as the result of evaluation process shall be restricted to an analysis of data that portray the total child.

11. Educational programming decisions shall be derived from data gathered from a variety of sources (e.g., in-school, home, com-

munity), and shall evolve from the synthesis of an interdisciplinary team effort. The parents shall be considered team members. When appropriate, the child shall be included.

12. Educational programming decisions shall be made on the basis
of individual student needs and behavioral strengths and weaknesses rather than on the child's handicapping condition.

STATEMENTS OF ASSUMPTIONS

- Aside from considerations of item bias, some tests give more reliable and valid information about a student than others; therefore,
some tests are more biased than others.
- The issue of bidialectism can be as great or greater than bilingualism and needs to be given the same consideration in the assessment process.
- It is unlikely that
  a. two individuals have had the same opportunity to learn the
     content, skills, and behaviors measured by assessment tools
  b. two individuals have been similarly rewarded for learning and
     are thus similarly motivated to learn
  c. two individuals are equally free of anxiety or emotional prob-
     lems that could interfere with learning or testing
  d. two individuals have had equal experience in the assessment
     process
  e. two developmentally disabled individuals are equally free of or
     equally affected by physical disability or sensory or motor
     handicaps that could interfere with learning.
- Inherent differences in innate abilities should be individually determined rather than being determined by sociocultural group
membership.
- Each individual is dynamic and fluid by nature, never remaining
static, and thus has the potential for measurable change.
- For each individual there are appropriate assessment techniques
and methods available to the assessment team.
- Members of the interdisciplinary team shall be advocates for the
student while acting in accordance with the ethical codes of their
individual professionals and adhering fully to the rules and regulations of the school system in which they are employed.
- Appropriate instructional programming requires skilled, knowledgeable examiners who consider the impact of sociocultural variables.

- The degree of bias in assessment must be controlled.
- Significant overlap exists between and across traditional cultures.
- Biased assessment is not exclusively a racial concern.
- No one should be assigned to special education unless his or her unique situation warrants such a placement.
- There is no individual who cannot be tested.
- Parents make a unique contribution to the assessment process and need to be intimately involved in each step.

ASSESSMENT PROCESS

The process itself is divided into six phases and 41 specific components indicating either an action step or a decision point. Phase I, problem identification, initiates the process which continues through pre-referral, referral, assessment, placement, and continuing evaluation. Emphasis is placed on the following items:

1. Pre-referral activities, which include a number of opportunities for dealing with the problem through regular education alternatives.
2. Numerous opportunities to discontinue the assessment process and refer the youngster back to an appropriate regular education environment.
3. Comprehensive assessment procedures which include traditional cognitive assessment as only one part of the total process.
4. Self-administered checklists and questionnaires to be completed at strategically selected points in the process to ensure that racial, cultural, or linguistic bias does not influence the educational decision.

Each box of the flow chart in Figure 4–2 represents one component or decision point of the assessment process and is supported by a corresponding process sheet. Process sheets describe the activities that take place during each step and provide a variety of other information, such as the persons responsible for implementation and cautions related to the implementation of the particular step. The specific location of the step is also depicted graphically with relation to the step(s) preceding and following in the process, as illustrated in Figure 4–3. Each step of the process is documented in precisely the same fashion.

Figure 4–2. PHASE 1. PROBLEM IDENTIFICATION

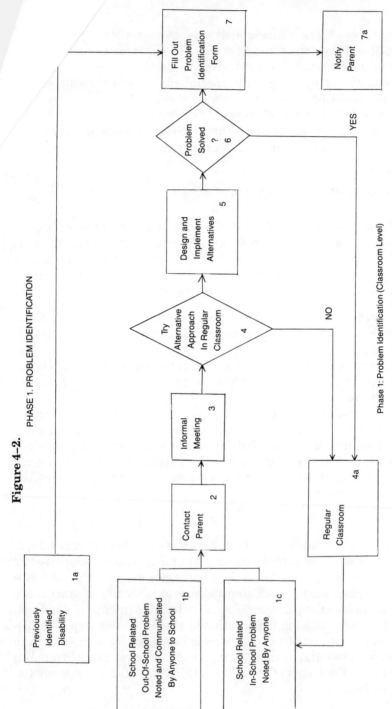

Phase 1: Problem Identification (Classroom Level)

PHASE 2: PRE-REFERRAL PROCESS (BUILDING LEVEL) REGULAR EDUCATION ALTERNATIVES

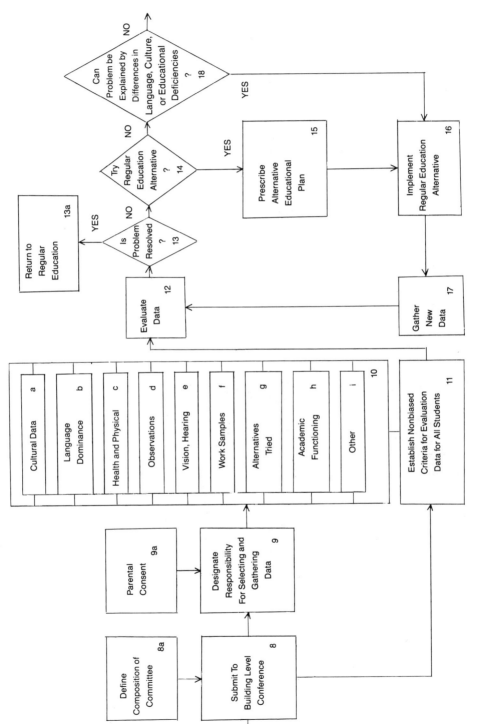

Figure 4–2 (continued)

PHASE 3: REFERRAL/ASSESSMENT (REGIONAL LEVEL)

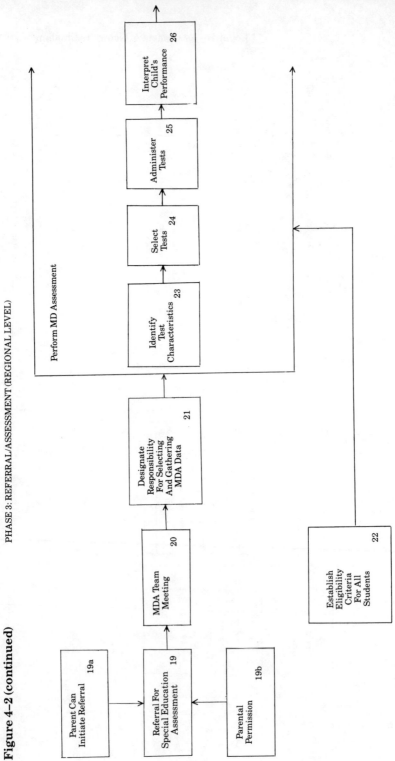

PHASE 3: REFERRAL/ASSESSMENT (REGIONAL LEVEL) — continued

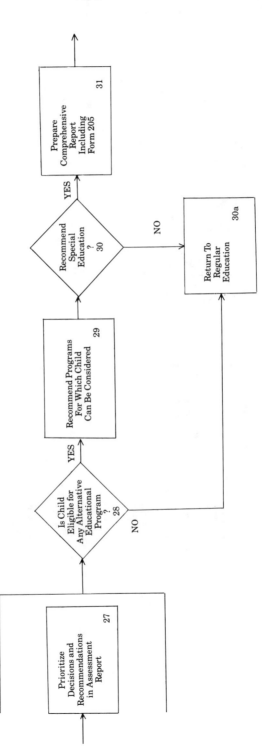

Figure 4-2 (continued)

PHASE 4: REFERRAL TO CHILD STUDY CENTER

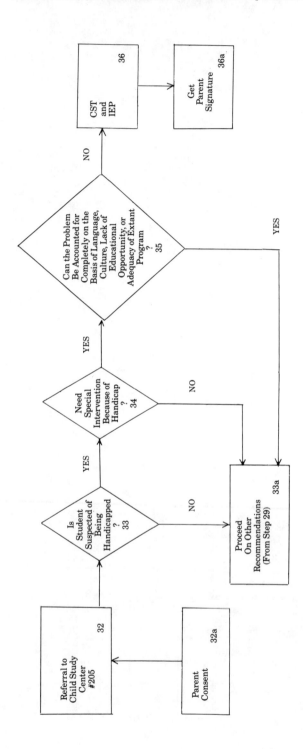

PHASE 5: PLACEMENT IN L.R.E.

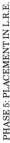

Select
Least
Restrictive
Environment

37

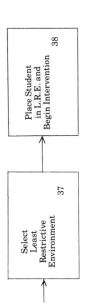

Place Student
in L.R.E. and
Begin Intervention

38

PHASE 6: CONTINUING EVALUATION

Evaluate
Student
Periodically

39

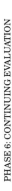

Perform
Annual Review
of Placement and
Progress and Make
Recommendations

40

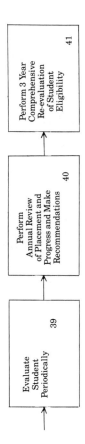

Perform 3 Year
Comprehensive
Re-evaluation
of Student
Eligibility

41

Figure 4–3.   PROCESS SHEET — Step 5

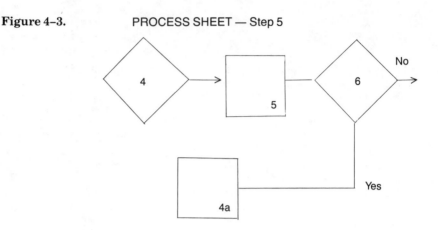

Title: Design and implement alternatives.

Person Responsible: Classroom teacher in conjunction with other staff members and parent if possible.

Process Overview: Appropriate school personnel (preferably the classroom teacher) designs and implements some alternative (classroom procedure) to regular classroom procedures, to help solve the child's problem.

Process Details:
1. The teacher asks a counselor for suggestions. The counselor designs strategies or alternatives that modify the child's environment either at home or school, such as the following:
   a. adjust child's schedule of classes,
   b. suggest different seating arrangement,
   c. recommend parent set up a study area in the home.
2. The teacher designs strategies or alternatives that modify the child's environment either at home or in school, such as the following:
   a. Change the reading program to see if child responds differently to another reading approach,
   b. suggest parent read with or to the child at home,
   c. set up a student-to-student tutoring program,
   d. change the structure or the routine of the day,
   e. give the child assistance in bilingual education,
   f. give the child assistance through another program, such as a Title I reading program.

Cautions:
1. When you choose alternatives be sure to think them through carefully. Don't automatically choose something because you think of it first. Consider how an alternative approach might affect the child.
2. Analyze your motives for selecting a particular approach. Does your approach have any discriminatory aspects (e.g., isolating the student from other class members)?
3. Try to include the parents in deciding on and designing the alternatives. The more they are involved actively from the beginning, the more helpful and accepting they will be if the pre-referral and referral processes continue. This means being actively involved in providing input, not passively involved (just being informed). You are initiating a parent-school partnership.

Next: Decision point: Has the problem been resolved at the classroom level? (Step 6)

Time and space restrictions do not allow for a more detailed presentation of the total assessment process. The scope of this chapter does, however, provide sufficient rationale for the inclusion of Steps 21 through 27 of Phase II, which contain that portion of the process wherein data are gathered from the variety of data sources. This portion of the assessment process, which traditionally includes evaluation of cognitive functioning, is referred to as the Multi-Disciplinary Assessment (MDA) (Figure 4–4). Note that the process is individualized for each child and that Steps 24, 25, 26, and 27 incorporate specific nondiscriminatory checklists that are designed to alert team members to potential sources of bias.

Figure 4–4.   PROCESS SHEET — Step 21

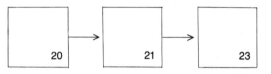

Title: Designate responsibility for selecting and gathering MDA data.

Person Responsible: Chairperson of MDA committee.

Process Overview: The chairperson in cooperation with the members of the MDA committee will determine what kind of information should be gathered and who should gather it.

Process Details:
1. The chairperson convenes a meeting of the committee to discuss the information already available on the child. Information gathered during pre-referral should be used and not duplicated unless there is a valid reason for suspecting the accuracy of the original data.
2. Based upon existing information and the child's problem, the committee should decide which additional information is needed.
3. The responsibility for gathering the different types of data should be assigned and time-lines established for the completion of assessment tasks.
4. Someone sensitive to the child's culture, mode of communication, handicapping condition, and language background should be a part of the assessment team and assist in gathering assessment data.
5. At this point, before doing any testing, the assessment team should discuss if any of the following could be influencing the child's problem in a primary manner:
    a. child's cultural background
    b. child's language background
    c. child's handicap
    d. child's mode of communication (oral, total, or manual)
6. It is necessary to include the parent as part of the assessment team whenever possible.
7. The following areas should be considered for assessment:
    a. language proficiency
    b. educational

Figure 4-4 (continued)

    c.   sensory-motor
    d.   adaptive behavior, social
    e.   medical
    f.   psychological, both intelligence and personality
    g.   vocational

Cautions:
1. The child's problem may be a result of absenteeism.
2. In order for the multidisciplinary team concept to work, different professionals must use their energies to build a trust relationship with other professionals, with mutual respect for each other's abilities and contributions to the assessment.
3. Care must be taken when testing a child who is bilingual, but whose dominant language is English. A monolingual psychologist may not be sensitive to relevant cultural differences even though the child and the psychologist share the same dominant language.

PROCESS SHEET — Step 22

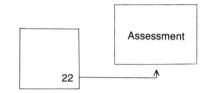

Title: Establish eligibility criteria for all students.

Persons Responsible: Multi-Disciplinary Assessment Committee.

Process: Before beginning the evaluation, establish appropriate criteria for evaluating the areas listed in Step 23. Criteria are defined levels of accomplishment on specific tests and measurement processes which can be applied during the evaluation process to provide standards for the judgment process.

If criteria are not established before the evaluation of a given child, the criticism can be raised that the criteria were chosen arbitrarily for the child being evaluated — hence the criteria may be biased and discriminatory.

Each test and evaluation procedure that is commonly used in the assessment process should be examined by an appropriate committee and minimal acceptable criteria are to be established for the population being served by the school.

Next Step: Perform MD assessment.

PROCESS SHEET — Step 23

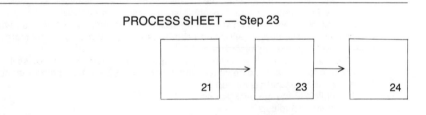

Title: Perform MDA Assessment — Identify test characteristics.

Person Responsible: Each professional in his or her field, as designated by the MDA team.

Process: Tests used in the MDA assessment should cover as broad a spectrum as possible, thereby yielding all important information about the child and his or her

Figure 4-4 (continued)

problem(s). Appropriate tests should be identified for each of the following evaluation areas:

Observational Data

Before a child is considered for special education programming, adequate information should be obtained from teachers and other educators who know the child and work directly with him or her. Such data should be required as support for the need for the referral. It is, in a sense, the child's first line of defense. Without such data, decision makers may act on the emotionally inspired requests of a single person who wants a child moved. When sufficient observational data accompany the initial consideration for special education, it is a relatively simple matter to prescribe immediate intervention that does not require further assessment.

Language Dominance Data

Determining the child's language dominance and the degree to which it is compatible with the language used in the school can be critical in determining the degree to which a child may or may not be exhibiting symptoms of a possible handicapping condition. Information on language dominance is needed primarily to avoid the misdiagnosis (and subsequent misplacement) of students who speak non-native English and to identify language deficiencies that need attention.

Educational Assessment Data

Under the available data section, general information about a child's academic progress was obtained. This information, however, may be an inaccurate reflection of the child's level of educational achievement or may be discrepant with the observational data reported with the referral. An in-depth, individually administered educational assessment is often necessary.

Sensory-Motor Assessment Data

The rationale is that sensory-motor difficulties are associated with learning handicaps and can be remedied, allowing for increase in learning.

Adaptive Behavior Data

It is important to know the degree to which behavior observed in the learning environment generalizes to other environments, such as the playground, the home, the neighborhood, and the community. Many children who do not function within normal limits in the traditional learning environment are quite capable of normal functioning in nonacademic settings.

Medical or Developmental Data

A child may show symptoms that appear to the casual observer to be evidence of a handicapping condition deserving special education intervention, when, in fact, the child is suffering from a medical problem that can be remedied by medical intervention. It is important to know the medical and developmental history of a child as well as current conditions when making decisions about educational programming.

Personality Assessment Data

Complex emotional and personality variables may interact to cause the child's referred behavior. It is quite helpful, therefore, to have valid data regarding these variables. The child may have no handicapping condition and his problem may be corrected by intervention strategies available through the regular school program. On the other hand, some form of psychosis or severe neurosis may be present and, if diagnosed, appropriate special education intervention can be provided. It is especially important to get the child's own viewpoint of the situation and how he or she perceives it by interviewing the child directly.

Intellectual Assessment Data

Tests of intellectual functioning are valuable tools that can provide objective, quantifiable, and predictive data regarding learning aptitudes. If we accept the perception that a basic role of the school is to foster academic development, these tests provide the best predictors of success. However, problems arise when the tests are used for the purpose of classifying students into ability levels for special education for the mentally retarded.

Figure 4-4 (continued)

Cautions:
 To understand the strengths and the limitations of the tests and other assessment
 procedures that you use, you must examine the following characteristics:
 a. How many items are there? Some tests have too few, some too many.
 b. What is the item content? Does it measure what you want it to?
 c. Is the child's behavior measured in the home or in the classroom, or is it
     generalized from the test setting?
 d. What languages are used on the test?
 e. In what alternate modes of communication is the test available?
 f. How adequate is the reliability?
 g. How adequate is the validity?
 h. What is the size and composition of the norm group?
Next Step: Select the tests to be used, Step 24.

PROCESS SHEET — Step 24

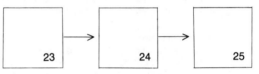

Title: Select tests.

Person Responsible: Each professional in his or her field, as designated by the MDA
 team.

Process: On the basis of information known about the child and the test data,
 appropriate tests and other measuring instruments and processes are selected.

Cautions:
 1. PL 94–142 encourages individualization in the selection of tests and assessment
     techniques. Therefore, have you matched the characteristics of the information
     needed on the child with the characteristics of and information generated by the
     test?
 2. Have you identified potential sources of bias with a particular test and decided
     how to minimize them?
 3. Have you used a combination of devices? The use of criterion-referenced
     devices and observation can supplement data from norm-referenced tests.
 4. Are you sure the test is appropriate for the purpose for which you are using it? If
     your purpose is placement, you must have data from some norm-referenced
     instrument.
 5. Have you selected more than one measure? Be sure measures are educationally
     sound and are relevant to all areas of suspected disability.

Nondiscriminatory Question Check
 1. Have I determined the best assessment approach for this child? _   ☐
 2. Considering the reasons for referral, do I need to utilize
     behavioral observations, interviews, informal techniques, or a
     combination of the above? _____   ☐
 3. Have I given as much thought to assessing this child's adaptive
     behavior as I have to his academic school performance? _____   ☐
 4. Are the approaches I am considering consistent with the child's
     receptive and expressive abilities? _____   ☐
 5. Am I placing an overdependence on one technique and
     overlooking others that may be more appropriate? _____   ☐
 6. Have I achieved a balance between formal and informal
     techniques in my selection? _____   ☐

Figure 4-4 (continued)

7. As I testing this child simply because I have always used tests in my assessment procedure? _____ ☐
8. Am I administering a particular test simply because it is part of "the battery"? _____ ☐
9. Am I administering a test because I have been directed to do so by the administration? _____ ☐
10. Does the instrument I have chosen include persons in the standardization sample from this child's cultural group? _____ ☐
11. Are subgroup scores reported in the test manual? _____ ☐
12. Were there large enough numbers of this child's cultural group in the test sample for me to have any reliance on the norms? _____ ☐
13. Does the instrument I have selected assume a universal set of experiences for all children? _____ ☐
14. Does the instrument selected contain illustrations that are misleading or outdated or not appropriate? _____ ☐
15. Does the instrument selected employ vocabulary that is colloquial, regional, or archaic? _____ ☐
16. Do I understand the theoretical basis of the instrument? _____ ☐
17. Will this instrument easily assist in delineating a recommended course of action to benefit this child? _____ ☐
18. Have I reviewed current literature regarding this instrument? ___ ☐
19. Have I reviewed current research related to potential cultural influences on test results? _____ ☐

Next Step: Administer the tests and evaluation processes, Step 25

PROCESS SHEET — Step 25

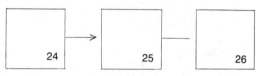

Title: Administer the tests.

Person Responsible: Each professional in his or her field, as designated by the MDA team.

Process: The tests which have been selected are administered.

Cautions: Have you checked for potential sources of bias in the following areas:
1. the examiner?
2. the testing situation or environment?
3. the interaction between the child and the examiner?
4. the order of subscales in a test or the order of tests in a battery? For example, a shy preschool child may not perform gross motor or expressive language tasks as well in the beginning of a testing situation as he or she would once he or she feels more comfortable.

Nondiscriminatory Question Check
1. Are there factors about the examiner that could bias the results (i.e., training, language mode, experiences testing similar types of children, attitudes toward particular cultural groups and about nonbiased assessment, and knowledge of alternative ways of giving tests)? _____ ☐
2. Could the physical environment of the testing setting adversely affect this child's performance (i.e., room temperature, noise, inadequate space, poor lighting, inappropriate furnishings, child size)? _____ ☐
3. Am I familiar with the test manual and have I followed its directions?_ ☐

Figure 4-4 (continued)

4. Have I given this child clear directions?_____   ☐
5. If the native language is not English, have I instructed him or her in
   his or her language?_____   ☐
6. Am I sure that this child understands my directions?_____   ☐
7. Have I accurately recorded entire responses to test items, even
   though the child's answers may be incorrect, so that I might later
   consider them when interpreting his or her test scores?_____   ☐
8. Did I establish and maintain rapport with this child throughout the
   evaluation session?_____   ☐
9. Did the child maintain attentive behavior throughout the session?__   ☐

Next Step: Interpreting the child's performance, Step 26.

PROCESS SHEET — Step 26

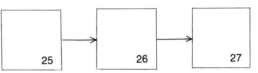

Title: Interpreting the child's performance.

Person Responsible: Each professional in his or her field, as designated by the MDA team.

Process: The child's performance on the tests and other evaluation instruments is interpreted in the light of test manuals, norms established on appropriate reference groups, and the criteria established in Step 22.

Cautions:
1. Have you examined, considered, and synthesized all of the collected information and uncovered potential sources of bias that could result in measurement error?
2. Have you compared results of multiple measures and sources and looked for similarities and differences?
3. How do these results compare to the measure of the child's adaptive behavior? A child must be delayed in both intellectual and adaptive behavior before he or she can be classified as mentally retarded.
4. What indications do you have that these results are representative of the child's behavior? For example, did you do more than one classroom observation?

Nondiscriminatory Question Check
1. Have you looked for characteristics of the child that might bias or
   influence the results, such as native language, age, health, nutrition,
   handicapping conditions, mode of communication, sensory and
   performance modalities, and emotional state? _____   ☐
2. Have you looked at the characteristics of the tests and techniques
   that might bias or influence the results, such as purpose,
   communication modalities, norms, reliability and validity, type of
   measure, relevance of items, scoring criteria, and type of scores? __   ☐
3. Have you looked at the characteristics of the examiners that might
   bias or influence the results, such as appropriate training,
   communication mode and language, previous experience, attitudes,
   skills, and knowledge? _____   ☐
4. Have you looked at the conditions within the assessment situation
   that might bias the performance, such as time of day, distractions,
   testing materials, inappropriate use of clues, length of session,
   comfort and accessibility of materials, and order of assessment
   activities? _____   ☐

Figure 4-4 (continued)

5. Have you looked for conditions between the examiners and child that might bias the performance, such as rapport, attending behavior, communication, directions, modeling or demonstrating, dress or mannerisms, and child's appearance? _____ ☐

Next Step: Prioritizing decisions and recommendations — Step 27.

PROCESS SHEET — Step 27

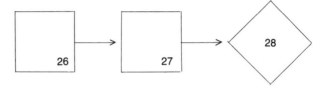

Title: Prioritizing decisions and recommendations: the assessment report.

Persons Responsible: The MDA team.

Process:
1. All information and data concerning the child is considered.
2. Alternative recommendations concerning the child are prepared.
3. The alternative recommendations are prioritized.
4. A formal report is prepared.

Nondiscriminatory Question Check
1. Is the report clearly written and free of educational jargon so that it can be easily understood by the child, parents, and teachers? _____ ☐
2. Does the report answer the questions asked in the referral? _____ ☐
3. Are the recommendations which have been made realistic and practical for the child, school personnel, teacher, and parents? _____ ☐
4. Has the committee provided alternative recommendations? _____ ☐
5. Does the report include a description of any problems that were encountered and the effects of such during the assessment process? _____ ☐

Next Step: Decide if the child is eligible for any alternative educational programs — Step 28.

SUMMARY

It has been argued successfully in the courts that the misclassification of minority children as mildly retarded is the result of overreliance on standardized IQ scores derived from individually administered tests of intelligence that are biased in favor of the majority population. In addition, questions have been raised with respect to the interpretation and use of such scores for the purpose of educational placement. The authors suggest that data derived from tests of intelligence can provide valid information concerning the extent to which a child has acquired the knowledge and thinking skills valued by the schools. These data have educational relevance only so long as they are used to measure current performance levels and not *innate potential.* They emphasize middle class values; hence, they are not culture-free. The diagnostician must expand the assessment process to determine fully the extent of a child's learning potential. An assessment process must be comprehensive in that it seeks out and uses data from a variety of sources, only one of which may be traditional assessment of cognitive function. An adequate and non-biased assessment process will include such areas as adaptive behavior, sociocultural factors, medical history, and so on. The alternative assessment strategies reviewed earlier (i.e., dynamic assessment) will also figure prominently in assessing any youngster's cognitive abilities.

REFERENCES

Blanton, R. L. (1975). Historical perspectives on classification of mental retardation. In N. Hobbs (Ed.), *Issues in the classification of children* (Vol. 1). San Francisco: Jossey-Bass.

Bogatz, B. E. (1976). *Proceedings of the national conference: With bias toward none.* Lexington: University of Kentucky.

Bogatz, B. E. (1977). *With bias toward none: A national survey of assessment programs and procedures.* Lexington: University of Kentucky.

Bogatz, B. E. (Ed.). (1981) *Procedural guidelines for non-discriminatory assessment in the public schools of the District of Columbia.* Washington, DC. (Unpublished.)

Brody, A. B., and Brody, N. (1976). *Intelligence, nature, determinants and consequences.* New York: Academic Press.

Brown v. Board of Education of Topeka. United States Supreme Court; 347 U.S. 483 (1954).

Budoff, M. (1972, June). Measuring learning potential: An alternative to the traditional intelligence test. In *Ethical and legal factors in the practice of school psychology. Proceedings of the First Annual Conference in School Psychology,* Temple University, Philadelphia.

Budoff, M., and Corman, L. (1976). Effectiveness of a learning potential procedure in improving problem-solving skills of retarded and nonretarded children. *American Journal of Mental Deficiency, 81,* 260–264.

Chinn, J. L. (1983). Diagnostic considerations in working with Asian-Americans. *American Journal of Orthopsychiatry, 53,* 100–109.

Crowner, J. (Ed.). (1980). *The Illinois registry of personnel with special skills in the assessment of bilingual/bicultural students and others with unique language needs.* Carbondale, IL: Department of Special Education, Southern Illinois University.

Dennis, W. (1942). The performance of Hopi children on the Goodenough Draw-a-Man Test. *Journal of Comparative Psychology, 34,* 341–348.

Diana v. California State Board of Education. United States District Court, Northern District of California, C-7037, RFP, 1969.

Dunn, L. M. (1968). Special education for the mildly retarded — is much of it justifiable? *Exceptional Children, 35,* 5–22.

Dunn, L. M. (1973). *Exceptional children in the schools: Special education in transition.* New York: Holt, Rinehart, and Winston.

Education of All Handicapped Children Act (1975). Public Law 94–142, November 29, 1975.

Federal Register (1977, Tuesday, August 23). Part II, Department of HEW: Office of Education, Education of Handicapped Children; Implementation of Part B of the Education of the Handicapped Act. Vol. *42,* W 163, 42474–42518.

Feuerstein, R. (1979). *The dynamic assessment of retarded performers.* Baltimore: University Park Press.

Feuerstein, R., and Rand, Y. (1977). Studies in cognitive modifiability: Redevelopment of cognitive function of retarded early adolescents. *Instrumental enrichment.* Jerusalem: Hadassah-Alizo — Canada Research Institute.

Flynn, J. R. (1983). Now the great augmentation of the American IQ. *Nature, 301,* 655.

Gould, S. J. (1981). *The mismeasure of man.* New York: W. W. Norton.

Guadalupe v. Tempe Elementary School District, Stipulation and Order (January 24, 1972).

Havighurst, R. J., Gunther, M. K., and Pratt, I. E. (1946). Environment and the Draw-a-Man Test: The performance of Indian children. *Journal of Abnormal and Social Psychology, 41,* 50–63.

Hobbs, N. (1974). *The futures of children: Categories, labels, and their consequences.* Nashville: Vanderbilt University.

Hobson v. Hansen, United States District Court. District of Columbia, 269 F. Supp. 4011 (B.D.C. 1967).

Jenson, A. (1969). How much can we boost IQ and scholastic achievement? *Harvard Education Review, 39,* 1–123.

Jones, R. L. (1972). Labels and stigma in special education. *Exceptional Children, 38,* 553–564.

Kamin, L. (1974). *The science and politics of IQ.* Potomac, MD: Erlbaum Associates.

Kaufman, A. S. (1979). *Intelligence testing with the WISC-R.* New York: John Wiley and Sons.

Kaufman, A.S., and Dappelt, J. E. (1976). Analysis of WISC-R standardization data in terms of the stratification variables. *Child Development,* 166–171.

Kuriloff, P. (1975). Law, education reform, and the school psychologist. *Journal of School Psychology, 13*(4), 335–348.

Larry P. v. Wilson Riles, No. C-71-2270 RFP, U.S. District Court for the Northern District of California. (October 16, 1979).

Larry P. v. Wilson Riles, No. CV 71-2270, United States Court of Appeals, Ninth Circuit. (January 23, 1984).

Lilly M. S. (1970). A teapot in a tempest. *Exceptional Children, 37,* 43–49.

Lilly, M. S. (1971). Training based model for special education. *Exceptional Children, 37,* 745–779.

Lynn, R. (1982). IQ in Japan and the United States shows a growing disparity. *Nature, 297,* 222–223.

Manni, J. L., Winikur, D. W., and Keller, M. (1984). *Intelligence, mental retardation, and the culturally different child.* Springfield, IL: Charles C Thomas.

Mercer, J. R. (1975). Psychological assessment and the rights of children. In N. Hobbs (Ed.), *Issues in the classification of children.* (Vol. 1) (pp. 130–159). San Francisco: Jossey-Bass.

Mercer, J. R. (1979). In defense of racially and culturally nondiscriminatory assessment. *School Psychology Digest, 8,* 89–115.

Mercer, J. R., and Lewis, J. F. (1977). *System of multicultural pluralistic assessment* (SOMPA). New York: Psychological Corporation.

Merton, R. K. (1948). The self-fulfilling prophecy. *Antioch Review, 8,* 193-210.

Messick, A. (1980). Test validity and the ethics of assessment. *American Psychologist, 35,* 1012–1027.

Naglieri, J. A., and Yazzie, C. (1983). Comparison of the WISC-R and PPVT-R with Navajo children. *Journal of Clinical Psychology, 39,* 598–600.

Oakland, T. (Ed.). (1976). *With bias toward none: Non-biased assessment of minority group children.* Lexington: University of Kentucky.

Oakland, T. (1979). Research on the adaptive behavior inventory for children and the estimated learning potential. *School Psychology Digest, 8,* 63–70.

Oakland, T. (1980). An evaluation of the ABOC, pluralistic norms, and estimated learning potential. *Journal of School Psychology, 18,* 34–11.

Parents in Action on Special Education (PASE) v. Joseph P. Hannon et al., No. 74C 3586, U.S. District Court for the Northern District of Illinois Eastern Division, 1980.

Portenier, L. C. (1945). Abilities and interests of Japanese-American high school seniors. *Journal of Social Psychology, 35,* 53–61.

Rehabilitation Act of 1973. Public Law 93–380.

Reschly, D. J. (1979). Nonbiased assessment. In G. Phye and D. J. Reschly (Eds.), *School psychology: Perspectives and issues.* New York: Academic Press.

Reschly, D. J. (1980). Psychological evidence in the Larry P. opinion: A case of right problem — wrong solution? *School Psychology Review, 9*(2), 123–135.

Rohrer, J. H. (1942). The test intelligence of Osage Indians. *Journal of Social Psychology, 16,* 99–105.

Rosenthal, R., and Jacobson, L. (1966). Teachers' expectancies: Determinants of pupils' IQ gains. *Psychological Reports, 19,* 115–118.

Sandiford, P., and Kerr, R. (1926). Intelligence of Chinese and Japanese children. *Journal of Educational Psychology, 17,* 361–387.

Sata, L. S. (1977). Musings of a hyphenated American. In S. Sue and N. N. Wagner (Eds.), *Asian Americans: Psychological perspectives.* Ben Lomond, CA: Science and Behavior Books.

Scarr, S. (1981). Testing for children: Assessment and the many determinants of intellectual competence. *American Psychologist, 36,* 1101, 1159–1171.

Shuey, A. (1966). *The testing of Negro intelligence.* New York: Social Science Press.

Smith, M. E. (1957). Progress in the use of English after 22 years in children of Chinese ancestry in Honolulu. *Journal of Genetic Psychology, 90,* 255–258.

Smith, M. E., and Kasdon, L. M. (1961). Progress in the use of English after 20 years by children of Filipino and Japanese ancestry in Hawaii. *Journal of Genetic Psychology, 99,* 129–178.

Stewart v. Phillips, 70-1199-F. (D. Mass. 1970).

Tucker, J. A. (1976). Operationalizing the diagnostic-intervention process. *With bias toward none: A national survey of assessment programs and procedures.* Lexington: University of Kentucky.

Vining, D. R., Jr. (1983). Mean IQ differences in Japan and the United States. *Nature, 301,* 738.

Wagner, N. N. (1977). Filipinos: A minority within a minority. In S. Sue and N. N. Wagner (Eds.), *Asian Americans: Psychological perspectives.* Ben Lomond, CA: Science and Behavior Books.

Wechsler, D. (1974). *Manual for the Wechsler Intelligence Scale for Children – Revised.* New York: Psychological Corporation.

Williams, R. L. (1974). From dehumanization to black intellectual genocide: A rejoinder. In G. J. Williams and S. Gordon (Eds.), *Clinical Child Psychology, Behavioral Publication* (pp. 320–323). New York.

Wilson, L. (1973). Canadian Indian children who had never attended school. *Alberta Journal of Educational Research, 14,* 309–313.

Wurtz, R. G. (1981). An investigation of the estimated learning potential and its ability to predict performance in experimental learning tasks. Doctoral dissertation, Temple University, 1981. *Dissertation Abstracts International, 42/12,* 4947 B.

Yoshioka, J. G. (1929). A study of bilingualism. *Pedagogical Seminary and Journal of Genetic Psychology, 36,* 473–479.

PART III
MANAGEMENT AND EDUCATIONAL ISSUES

Chapter 5

Clinical Principles for Language Intervention Among Nonstandard Speakers of English

Harry N. Seymour

Historically, an almost exclusive research and clinical focus on speakers of standard English dialects has left a formidable gap in knowledge of clinical strategies for speakers of nonstandard dialects. Because dialectal variation in the United States is great and mirrors a socially diverse populace (Allen and Underwood, 1971; McDavid and McDavid, 1951; Toliver-Weddington, 1979; Wolfram and Fasold, 1974), social and cultural factors must be considered in the clinical process. To do otherwise ignores important factors that are unique to speakers of different dialects and impedes effective delivery of clinical services.

Clearly there is a need for greater understanding of dialect differences and for a clinical perspective that appropriately addressed these differences. However, the adoption of a dialectal perspective need not imply dramatically different clinical methods for every dialect. Instead, the clinician should modify methods according to pertinent sociolinguistic factors but not alter fundamental clinical principles that would prevail regardless of the dialect involved. Thus, the purpose of this chapter is to propose principles upon which clinical intervention strategies may be established for children who are language disordered and who are also of nonstandard English backgrounds.

CLINICAL PRINCIPLES

Six principles are identified as important for clinical intervention with children of nonstandard English backgrounds. These principles assert that intervention strategies represent language models that are (1) multidimensional, (2) interactive, (3) generative, (4) child-centered, (5) bidialectal, and (6) diagnostic. The principles delineate concepts the author considers necessary for effective clinical management of language disorders with children of nonstandard English backgrounds. The importance of these principles lies in their role in language learning, which is discussed later in this chapter, along with clinical implications.

Multidimensional Model

During the past decade or so, an explosion of information on language acquisition has led to a greater awareness of the multidimensional nature of language. In this respect, a major thrust has been directed toward the relationship between language structure and function. Structural aspects of language refer to the sounds that make up words (phonemes), words and inflections (morphemes), and word order (syntax). Language function refers to the complex interaction between meaning and communicative intent of a speaker. Although structure and function can be discussed and analyzed separately, they are multidimensional, interdependent, and inextricably bound when communicating through language.

A greater understanding of the relationship between structure and function has resulted in large part from the work of linguists, particularly psycholinguists and sociolinguists. Their work bridges the gap between the child's ability to understand language and his or her ability to use language. Although some linguists devote their attention to the structural framework of language, others, the psycholinguists, attempt to identify the psychological processes underlying the decoding and encoding of ideas represented by linguistic symbols. Still others, the sociolinguists, ponder how language use is influenced by both linguistic and nonlinguistic context.

Also, in recent years, psycholinguists have directed much attention to the relationship between cognition and language. Although this relationship is not altogether clear, the prevailing notion is that normal cognitive development is crucial to normal language development. Some argue that cognition is the foundational underpinning for language (Muma, 1978). This underpinning may be characterized by highly predictable cognitive milestones through which children pass that directly affect language (Bruner, 1975; Piaget, 1970; Sinclair-DeZwart, 1969).

During the sensorimotor period, the appearance of cognitive behaviors such as anticipation, causality, delayed imitation, and object permanence precede certain language milestones and may indicate language readiness for those milestones (Piaget, 1970). As the child grows older and passes from an iconic-imagery bound cognitive state to symbolic reasoning, his or her language behavior is still affected by cognitive constraints. Reliance on perceptual imagery and the "here and now" for processing information is reflected in cognitive behaviors such as failure to do conservation tasks and multiple-classification operations. These cognitive limitations show up in language behavior, as evidenced by overextensions. Language and cognition mirror developmental patterns that appear to be inextricably linked. Through cognition children process information about the world around them, which becomes the semantic foundation for language behavior. Indeed, language is a means for expressing what the child knows; what the child knows is determined by cognition. It is unlikely that a child learning the word "truck" first learns the label and then proceeds to find something with which to associate that label. Instead, there is evidence that children first process information about objects and events in their environment and then determine what they are called (Bloom, 1973; Bowerman, 1973; Nelson, 1973).

Although not without exception, this pattern of learning word meanings illustrates the foundational influence of cognition on language development. Thus, speech-language pathologists must consider the child's cognitive behaviors as well as language behaviors in diagnosing and treating language disorders.

Another major impact on how language should be viewed by speech-language pathologists has come from sociolinguists. Clearly, the use of language is a social phenomenon. According to Miller (1973), language is a "socially shared means for expressing ideas." Humans use language in social contexts for cooperative efforts, need fulfillment, knowledge acquisition, and manipulation. In fact, the primary motivation behind language functioning may be the individual's need to control and manipulate the environment. As such, it is social context that greatly influences what and how language is performed and represents a major domain of interest for sociolinguists.

According to sociolinguistic theory, context and language function greatly determine what is said and how it is said (Bates, 1976; Dore, 1975; Labov, 1970). Language context is both linguistic and nonlinguistic. The linguistic context is the form of language used in the speaking situation, and the nonlinguistic context is represented by the social context in which the discourse takes place. The form of the language varies as a function of the nonlinguistic context in which it is spoken.

Language function refers to the interpersonal (pragmatic) and intrapersonal (mathetic) bases for using language, that is, the speaker's communicative intent. This communicative intent may be represented by speech acts such as greeting, comment, rejection, denial, question, and so forth (Dore, 1975). Obviously there is interdependency among communicative intent, and linguistic and nonlinguistic contexts.

Aspects of language function and context may be observed very early in the language behavior of children. Halliday's observations (1977) about his son Nigel point out the early emergence of inter- and intrapersonal dimensions of language. As young as 13 months of age, Nigel used language interpersonally to fulfill his needs by *regulating* and *manipulating* others, and intrapersonally for *personal* and *heuristic* gratification. These behaviors reflect Nigel's need to communicate, which may be viewed as an extremely powerful motivation for learning language.

The perspectives of both sociolinguists and psycholinguists add to our understanding of language and its development. Of course, all linguists, to some degree, describe the form or structure of the language — what children learn when they learn language. However, sociolinguists offer insight into the motivation behind language learning — why children talk. In addition, psycholinguists answer questions about the underlying psychological processes in language learning — how children learn language. These points of view are mutually compatible and collectively contribute to the understanding of child language acquisition.

Given the various perspectives discussed earlier, it is important for the speech-language pathologist to approach speech and language problems in a multidimensional way. The roles of language structure, cognition, context, and function must be considered. In recent years, various authors have attempted to address this issue. Muma (1978) writes of *linguistic-cognitive-communicative* dimensions in describing language; Bloom and Lahey (1978) proposed a three-dimensional view of language, constituting *form-content-use.* These authors, as well as others, are attempting to define the most important aspects of language as a cognitive-content dimension, represented by concepts; a structural-form dimension, represented by phonology, syntax, and morphology; and a language use dimension, represented by pragmatics and mathetics. This model is depicted in Figure 5-1.

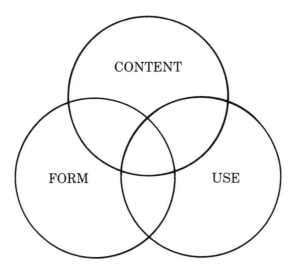

Figure 5-1. Interaction among content, form, and use. After Bloom, L., and Lahey, M. (1978). *Language development and language disorders.* New York: Wiley.

A multidimensional view of language, such as the form-content-use format, is of considerable value in language intervention generally, and most particularly with nonstandard English speakers (Seymour and Miller-Jones, 1981). Because so many of the forms of nonstandard English would be considered omission and substitution patterns in standard English, it is useful and necessary to look beyond form to understand the dialectal nature of these patterns. For example, a child who omits the -*s* plurality marker may be doing so for reasons of dialect, developmental immaturity, or pathology. To discern which of these possible causes is correct, the clinician must go beyond the form representation of the marker to a level of meaning (content) in which a child's understanding of the concept of plurality may be determined. Hence, questions about whether a child understands the underlying meaning (content) of a linguistic feature (form) and displays this understanding in appropriate contexts (use) is most revealing about that child's language functioning.

Intervention strategies for nonstandard English speaking children must be multidimensional even though most linguistic descriptions about nonstandard English center on form exclusively. Current literature, however, suggests little difference between standard English and nonstandard English in aspects other than form

(Brown, 1973; Seymour and Seymour, 1981; Slobin, 1979; Stockman and Vaughn-Cooke, 1981). Whether this contention is correct requires further research. Nevertheless, the speech-language pathologist must not focus solely on the child's form to the exclusion of meaning (content) and communicative intent (use).

Interactive Model

Given the view that language behavior is multidimensional, it follows that form, content, and use, as the major dimensions of language, are interdependent and interactive. No meaningful speech event can take place without these dimensions occurring simultaneously. The form of language (phonemes, morphemes, and syntax) is meaningless without content (concepts); both form and content are without purpose in the absence of use (communicative intent). Thus, because language is acquired in a multidimensional and interactive manner, language intervention should also be, if at all possible, multidimensional and interactive.

The position is taken here that when any single dimension of language is focused on to the exclusion of others, a less than optimal learning milieu is created. If a clinician attempts to facilitate language in a context devoid of meaning and communicative intent, the methods are likely to be artificial, contrived, and noninteractional. The methods that focus on target language behaviors, out of meaningful context, typically involve repetitive drills. Such methods are the least conducive for learning language because they lack mutual support and reinforcement among language structure (form), meaning (content), and intent (use). In contrast, language taught within meaningful contexts draws on the support that meaning gives to form and intent gives to meaning. Moreover, there may be a reinforcing quality to producing language purposefully and being understood.

Intervention goals that reflect an interactional model will include as many dimensions as possible. The more meaningful the context in which goals are to be implemented, the greater the opportunity and necessity for interaction among dimensions. Of course, the nature of the child's problem greatly determines the extent to which goals can be multidimensional and interactive. For example, a hyperactive and inattentive child will probably need a highly structured context involving narrowly focused goals. However, as the child progresses, the clinician should be ever conscious of the need to foster goals that stimulate a learning context that is meaningful and communicatively natural.

Generative Model

A generative model of language behavior refers to the capacity of humans to generate language spontaneously, creatively, and with infinite variety. According to the theory of generative grammar (Chomsky, 1957, 1965) humans are capable of generating language from a set of rules that constitute a grammar. The term grammar, as used here, does not refer to the "grammar" of the English teacher (i.e., the grammarian). Instead of meaning rules for the production of correct sentences, grammar is an abstract concept that pertains to underlying rules for the generation of meaningful language. The linguist views grammar as an hypothesis about the knowledge that makes a person a speaker of a language, not as a rigidly narrow prescription of what is considered "correct."

The concept of generative grammar has played an important role in child language acquisition theory. Although there are other prominent theories, generative grammar has helped clarify what it is that children acquire when they acquire language. Its basic tenet is that children unconsciously learn a finite set of linguistic rules that allow for the infinite generation of novel utterances (Chomsky, 1957, 1965). These rules are acquired early and somewhat effortlessly. By the age of approximately 4 or 5 years, most children have mastered their grammar. Of course, there are subtle aspects still to be acquired, but it is generally agreed that the basic grammar is present (Dale, 1976).

The ability to generate language from a finite grammar represents the *competence* that all speakers of a language possess. The acquisition of this competence is a universal human trait. Regardless of the country, the language, or the dialects that constitute a language, normal children of all races and socioeconomic statuses acquire the language to which they are exposed. Although many different dialects are spoken within the United States, some of which are standard and some nonstandard, these dialects have in common the basic grammar of English. (A basic grammar may be thought of as the knowledge common to speakers of different dialects of the same language.) For this reason, speakers of one dialect should not be considered linguistically inferior to speakers of other dialects because competence as speakers of English is not specific to any one dialect (Labov, 1970, 1972).

Consider the following negative forms:

1. I ain't got none.
2. I don't got none.

3. I don't have any.
4. I have none.

Each of these sentences is characteristic of a different dialect and contrasts in surface-structure representation. Speakers of these sentences may be thought of as being different in how they produce negative sentences, but not different in their ability to understand the concepts of negation represented by these contrasting sentences. This understanding exists because in addition to the *surface structure* of an utterance, there is a *deep structure* in which the meaning of that utterance is evident. As indicated in the examples given, there may be many surface representations for the same deep structure meaning. Even though these various negative forms represent different dialects, the speakers are nevertheless mutually understandable because they all speak a form of English.

Also represented by the differences among these negative sentences is a "performance-competence" contrast. Although an individual's language performance is a reflection of his or her language competence, the relationship is not isomorphic (Slobin, 1979). Because of sociolinguistic reasons, speakers can differ in how they express identical concepts of negation (performance) and yet all be competent. Moreover, in addition to this sociolinguistic basis for performance differences, competent language users may differ for psycholinguistic reasons as well. The emotional and physical state of the speaker can certainly affect performance. Indeed, it would be irrational to think that an individual is incompetent in language because of a slip of tongue, a forgotten word, a hesitation, or whatever aspect of language performance that may be momentarily and situationally deviant.

Thus, the generative model establishes a normal profile for language users that takes into account performance differences, either sociolinguistic or psycholinguistic in nature. The implications of this model for the speech-language pathologist are important. In determining language pathology, the clinician cannot have as a referent for normalcy surface structures that simply represent performance factors and not deep structure competency.

The implication of the generative model is to evaluate not only the form of what a speaker says but also the underlying meaning. The important question is whether the speaker is competent. To answer this question the clinician must discern what the speaker knows about the grammar of his or her language. This speaker knowledge is reflected in the ability to generate language appropriate to the situation and context. And, although the structure or form is important, it may be secondary to the overall communication of meaning. It must be kept in mind that if a speaker has acquired a language normally, that speaker has competence — a grammar that allows for the generation of infinite possibilities in communicating meaning. Hence, the speech-language pathologist must determine whether and how well the child has acquired the grammar of his or language.

How well a child has acquired a grammar can only be inferred because knowledge of a grammar is unconscious and intuitive. The knowledge an individual has about the rules of language is not conscious. Instead, it is tacit, intuitive, and unconscious. Just as a person knows how to tie shoes simply and easily, most speakers of a language know the rules of their language but have difficulty describing those rules, as they would have difficulty describing the process of tying their shoe laces.

Of course, language rules can be transformed from intuitive knowledge to reflective knowledge. The diagram of the sentence *The dog chased the cat* illustrates how a sentence composition can be made reflective.

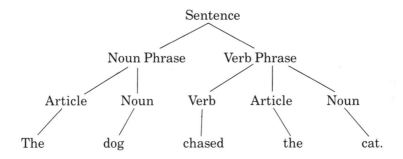

The diagramming of a sentence into constituent parts represents knowledge that reflects back on itself or mirrors the very knowledge that makes the sentence possible. Most speakers do not have this kind of reflective knowledge for the variety and complex sentence structures they routinely utter. They nevertheless know the rules (grammar), as is evidenced by their ability to speak the language.

Thus, the clinician has the difficult task of determining a child's competency with a grammar that cannot be observed directly. Clients generally are not asked to demonstrate their reflective knowledge, and even if they were, they could not. So, the clinician must rely on the child's communicative performance to make inferences about competence. These inferences are best made from observations of children's ability to generate language in a variety of communicative contexts.

The key term here is *generate*. Too often, speech-language pathologists attempt to determine the nature of pathology by assessing children's ability to perform a number of artificial tasks removed from the communicative context. In contrast, the generative model encourages assessment of children's abilities in a social and dynamic way, so that inferences are made more validly about their competence in communicating through language. Hence, intervention strategies focus on the child's competence in generating language in meaningful communicative contexts, as opposed to drills and exercises that are devoid of such meaning.

The generative model establishes a logical frame of reference for intervention with children speaking nonstandard English. It reflects a perspective that tolerates linguistic diversity wherein differences among speakers are considered natural and expected. Whether these differences are sociolinguistic or psycholinguistic, they constitute legitimate variations. On the other hand, toleration for variance does not include abnormalities of language, which is evident when an individual is incapable or has difficulty communicating ideas. This difficulty results from an inadequate acquisition of a grammar or a handicapping condition that prevents the use of language in a normal communicative way. Thus, the model of generative grammar is an important concept for language intervention and establishes a philosophical orientation for the clinician.

Child-Centered Model

Typically, plans for language intervention represent attempts to follow the language developmental schedules of normal children (Bloom and Lahey, 1978). Such an approach is reasonable and effective to the extent that the course of language development is known. However, the "state of the art" with respect to milestones of language development reflects considerable gaps. And, although normative profiles of language milestones are informative as guides, they nevertheless represent averages in the development of language forms that can vary by as much as 18 months (Prutting, 1979). Indeed, the rate, and to a lesser degree, the sequence, of language acquisition is extremely variable among children.

Given the limitations in knowledge about language acquisition and the variability among children, it is a most difficult task to establish with confidence a language impaired child's language level relative to that of other children of his or her peer group and to determine the language learning plan for intervention goals. This task is difficult at best when working with the child of standard English background for whom there exists language developmental data. But for the child of a nonstandard English background, about whom there is little developmental data (Seymour and Miller-Jones, 1981; Vaughn-Cooke, 1983), the determination of a language level based on developmental norms is highly questionable.

In considering alternative strategies for establishing language learning plans for the nonstandard English-speaking child, it is informative to consider two important facts about language learning behavior generally. The first is the synergistic nature of language learning. Children do not appear to learn forms in an additive and all-or-none manner. For example, they do not learn present progressive -*ing*, master that form, and then proceed to master the next form. Instead, the child is learning language synergistically, with many forms being acquired simultaneously under conditions of cognitive and linguistic constraints.

Figure 5–2 is an adaptation from a child language developmental schema taken from Crystal, Fletcher, and Garmen (1976). This figure shows a hypothetical progression for the learning of language in which a child passes through stages of development. Each stage is marked by a dominant language characteristic for which the stage is identified. For purposes of illustration, these stages simply are characterized by the acquisition of one, two, three, and four word elements, respectively. Thus, the child's language patterns are dominated by the one word element in Stage I. But, at the same time, there are utterances of at least two words found in his or her speech, as reflected in the overlapping of Stage I's curve into Stage II. In Stage II, the child's length of utterance is dominated by two words, but there are three and four word elements present, as well as one word elements of the previous Stage I. By Stage III, the child is using three words predominantly, but also has one, two and four word elements.

What Figure 5–2 shows is an unfolding of language that is synergistic. While the child is mastering certain forms, others are emerging, and earlier forms, not yet mastered, continue to exist. Thus, in keeping with the hypothetical four stages depicted in Figure 5–2, a child in Stage III, as an example, could be producing three word elements 60 percent of the time, four word elements 30 percent of the time, two word elements 20 percent of the time, and one word elements 10 percent of the time. This synergistic unfolding of language must be taken into consideration in language intervention.

The second important factor is variability of children in acquir-

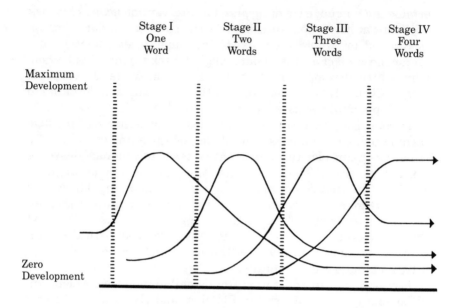

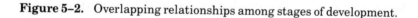

Figure 5–2. Overlapping relationships among stages of development.

ing language. As was evident by the foregoing example, there is variability within the child's language system. There is also variability among children (Bloom, Lightbown, and Hood, 1975). This variability among children is caused by many factors, not the least of which are cognitive and linguistic constraints associated with differing maturational schedules. Cognitive and linguistic constraints cause children to use different strategies in learning language and to learn at different rates.

These two factors, synergism and variability, are of major importance in establishing intervention goals for the language impaired child. Recognition of the synergistic and variable nature of language development should discourage speech-language pathologists from blindly following developmental profiles without regard for the individual child's emerging system. Thus, it seems unreasonable to establish 100 percent production goals for each of a succession of language forms when children acquire language in a synergistic and nonadditive manner. Moreover, the establishment of intervention goals for a sequence of development that presumably fits all children denies the variability that is known to exist.

Because language development is synergistic and variable, the only practical approach to describing a child's language problem is to individualize the process (i.e., take a child-centered approach). This may be done by establishing goals based on a within-subject analysis rather than based on group norms. A within-subject analysis focuses on the child's level of language knowledge without regard to how the child ranks in terms of group norms. With such an approach, group developmental norms would be used merely as a guide and put into perspective relative to the individual child's language system. Hence, each child is considered a "puzzle" for which solutions require information that is sufficient for making reasonable hypotheses about that child's competency.

The child-centered model is most suited for the nonstandard English speaking child. Because there is the issue of nonstandard English, in addition to concerns about synergistic development and variability, the child of a nonstandard English background presents a challenging "puzzle." The solution to this puzzle is to identify the child's strengths and weaknesses, which provides the basis for establishing intervention goals. This is achieved through an analysis of each child's emerging system and a determination of which forms he or she is and is not capable of using within a multidimensional, interactive, and generative frame of reference.

Bidialectal Model

Nontandard dialects of American English are marked by certain linguistic features that make them less acceptable than standard English dialects. The basis for this bias is often educational achievement (Edwards, 1979). Standard English tends to be spoken by the more educated of the society, and thus has a higher prestige value. However, the linguistic forms that differentiate the dialects are few in number and are relatively superficial (Labov, 1972; Wolfram, 1983). Even for a nonstandard dialect such as Black English vernacular, which differs more from standard English than other dialects, the similarities with standard English in structural form are far greater than the differences (Burling, 1973).

Of more significance than the surface structural differences between nonstandard and standard dialects is that they apparently have the same deep structure. There are no concepts that can be expressed in one dialect that cannot be expressed in another, even though there are idiosyncratic differences. And, for the most part, speakers of one dialect have relatively little difficulty in understanding speakers of another dialect. Where cross-dialectal unintelligibility is likely to occur is when standard English speakers have difficulty understanding nonstandard English speakers (Baran and Seymour, 1976; Nober and Seymour, 1979), but rarely does the reverse occur.

Minor intelligibility problems notwithstanding, speakers of varieties of English dialects, both standard and nonstandard, may be thought of as bidialectal to some degree. Of course this bidialectism does not necessarily mean that the nonstandard English speaker can speak standard English, or vice versa, even though there is mutual understanding. Yet, most speakers of nonstandard English do in fact have some degree of facility in speaking standard English. This facility is most apparent when speakers switch in an alternating fashion from linguistic characteristics of one dialect to those of another (Ratusnik and Koenigsknecht, 1975). Alternations of this kind, referred to as code switching, are most indicative of a bidialectal continuum between standard English and nonstandard English (Seymour and Seymour, 1977).

Indeed, the relationship between standard and nonstandard dialects may be viewed as an overlapping continuum in which there is an extension in knowledge from standard to nonstandard English features and a pattern of code switching between the two dialects. Because of the stigmatized nature of nonstandard English features, code switching is most likely to occur in one direction (i.e., from nonstandard to standard English forms).

Code switching represents the optional use of certain linguistic form. This use is determined by optional rules as opposed to obligatory rules. Rules that are obligatory require the occurrence of a particular form in a particular linguistic context. An example of an obligatory rule in standard English would be the -*s* plural marker. This form is optional in Black English in that it may be either deleted or produced, as evidenced by the following contrast, *The boy has two books → The boy has two book.* Optional rules also occur in standard English as in the case of contractible copula *He is tall → He's tall.* Although this contraction is also an option in nonstandard dialects, in Black English vernacular speakers may delete this form altogether (*He tall*).

The significance of optional rules is that features vary for a reason — they are not random occurrences. Optionality in the use of forms varies according to certain constraints, most notably linguistic and social. The linguistic constraints are those that facilitate the use of a particular feature. In the case of -*s* morpheme marker, there is a higher probability that speakers of Black English vernacular will use this form in expressing plurality (*He has two book*[*s*]) than in third person subject verb agreement (*The boy walk*[*s*] *home*). In this example, the grammatical rule for third person subject verb agreement is a stronger Black English vernacular rule than is plurality marker (Wolfram and Fasold, 1974). Similarly, past tense -*ed*, for example, will occur far more frequently in a phonemic environment such as *He play(ed) animal trainer* than in *He play(ed) basketball.* Because of abutting consonants between *played* and *basketball,* the consonant cluster reduction rule encourages the deletion of past tense -*ed*. Hence, there are linguistic constraints that encourage the existence of a form in one linguistic environment and not in others.

Social constraints refer to those nonlinguistic factors that increase the probability of nonstandard English usage. Race, socioeconomic status, and educational achievement are among social constraints that interact within a speaking context to influence the use of nonstandard English features. Also, the stigmatized nature of nonstandard English places demand upon speakers to use standard English in certain situations and not in others (Labov, 1970). Indeed, there is considerable pressure on Black children to use standard English in the school setting. At the same time, there is an opposing pressure from peers to use nonstandard English to maintain cohesive cultural identity and unity. As a consequence of educational demands for standard English and the counter demands for nonstandard English, children inevitably code switch.

The implications of bidialectism and code switching for the speech-language pathologist are considerable. A clinician must consider code switching to effectively assess and correct language problems among nonstandard English speakers. An understanding of code switching behavior is necessary for the correct identification and description of pathological behavior and to establish situational and linguistic contexts conducive for effective intervention. Further elaboration of these points will be made in Chapter 6.

Diagnostic-Intervention Model

Language intervention goals represent a learning plan for improving aspects of language behavior. This intervention plan is typically based on diagnostic information, and therefore the relationship between language diagnosis and intervention is an interdependent one. The interdependence begins with the diagnostic plan and continues throughout the intervention period. The continuous nature of the relationship between diagnosis and intervention becomes clear when we consider what the clinician must accomplish in the diagnostic process.

In diagnosis, the clinician attempts to answer three questions: (1) Does the child have a problem? (2) What is the nature of the problem? (3) What should the intervention goals be? The first question, regarding the existence of a problem, is answered by establishing that the child's speech or language behavior is sufficiently different from that of peers to warrant intervention. To this end, direct observations, language sampling, information from referral sources, medical records, and home and school behavioral history are helpful. Once this question is answered to the clinician's satisfaction, the more difficult task — answering the second question, about the nature of the problem — is tackled. The speech-language pathologist must now devise means by which to assess the child's "competency" (i.e., the child's level of language knowledge).

What a child knows about his or her language can be assessed only through what he or she does. Of course, what he or she does is "performance," and, as was discussed under Principle 3 (Generative Model), performance may not always accurately reflect competence. Consequently, the clinician is in the position of formulating hypotheses and testing these hypotheses, recognizing full well that results obtained are inferences about the child's competence. Inferences are not objective facts, but estimates of the child's language level.

Because intervention goals are based on inferences they should not be "etched in stone." Instead, these goals should be tentative plans subject to revision. There are two important reasons for this tentativeness. First, as noted earlier, the plan is an estimate, and thus it should be changed in response to new information. Second, the status of the client's language will continually change because it is still an emerging system, developing in response to maturational and social factors. The child's language is in a state of flux, subject to somewhat unpredictable changes in response to internal factors and external stimuli, of which clinical intervention is a part. Hence, as the language system unfolds, the language learning plan must correspondingly adapt.

The position that intervention goals reflect an ongoing diagnostic process may be viewed as a form of *diagnostic intervention*. The initial few hours following a diagnosis cannot possibly yield the kind of information necessary to determine valid intervention goals. The speech-language pathologist must accept a degree of ambivalence as goals are formulated, tested, and revised — all while simultaneously attempting to facilitate language learning.

SUMMARY

Six clinical principles considered important for effective language intervention with children of nonstandard English backgrounds are identified in this chapter. These principles hold that intervention strategies should be based on a learning plan that is (1) multidimensional, (2) interactional, (3) generative, (4) bidialectal, (5) child-centered, and (6) diagnostic. The rationale behind these principles is that they either are essential factors in the language learning process or represent factors particularly relevant to the nonstandard English speaking child. These six clinical principles form a theoretical framework for the author's proposed intervention strategies, presented in Chapter 6.

REFERENCES

Allen, H. B., and Underwood, G. N. (1971). *Readings in American dialectology.* New York: Appleton-Century-Crofts.

Baran, J., and Seymour, H. N. (1976). The influence of three phonological rules of Black English on the discrimination of minimal word pairs. *Journal of Speech and Hearing Research, 1,* 467–474.

Bates, E. (1976). Pragmatics and sociolinguistics in child language. In D. Morehead and A. Morehead (Eds.), *Normal and deviant child language* (pp. 411–463). Baltimore: University Park Press.

Bloom, L. (1973). *One word at a time: the use of single-word utterances before syntax.* The Hague, Netherlands: Mouton.

Bloom, L., and Lahey, M. (1978). *Language development and language disorders.* New York: Wiley.

Bloom, L., Lightbown, P., and Hood, L. (1975). Structure and variation in child language. *Monographs of the Society for Research in Child Development, 40,* 160.

Bowerman, M. (1973). Structural relationships in children's utterances: syntactic or semantic? In T. Moore (Ed.), *Cognitive development and the acquisition of language* (pp. 197–213). New York: Academic Press.

Brown, R. (1973). *A first language.* Cambridge, MA: Harvard University Press.

Bruner, J. (1975). The ontogenesis of speech acts. *Journal of Child Language, 2,* 1–19.

Burling, R. (1973). *English in black and white.* New York: Holt, Rinehart and Winston.

Chomsky, N. (1957). *Syntactic structures.* The Hague, Netherlands: Mouton.

Chomsky, N. (1965). *Aspects of the theory of syntax.* Cambridge, MA: MIT Press.

Crystal, D., Fletcher, P., and Garman, M. (1976). *The grammatical analysis of language disability.* New York: Elsevier.

Dale, P. (1976). *Language development: Structure and function* (2nd ed.). New York: Holt, Rinehart and Winston.

Dore, J. (1975). Holophrases, speech acts, and language universals. *Journal of Child Language, 2,* 21–40.

Edwards, J. R. (1979). *Language and disadvantage.* Amsterdam: Elsevier.

Halliday, M. A. (1977). *Explorations in the functions of language.* London: Arnold.

Labov, W. (1970). *The logic of non-standard English.* In F. Williams (Ed.), *Language and Poverty.* Chicago: Markham.

Labov, W. (1972). *Language in the inner city.* Philadelphia: University of Pennsylvania Press.

McDavid, R., and McDavid, V. (1951). The relationship of the speech of American Negroes to the speech of whites. *American Speech, 26,* 3–17.

Miller, G. (1973). *Communication, language, and meaning: Psychological perspectives.* New York: Basic Books, Inc.

Muma, J. (1978). *Language handbook, concepts, assessment, intervention.* Englewood Cliffs, NJ: Prentice-Hall.

Nelson, K. (1973). Some evidence for the cognitive primacy of categorization and its functional basis. *Merrill-Palmer Quarterly, 19,* 21–39.

Nober, E. H., and Seymour, H. N. (1979). Speaker intelligibility of Black and White school children for Black and White adult listeners under varying listening conditions. *Language and Speech, 22,* 237–242.

Piaget, J. (1970). Piaget's theory. In P. Mussen (Ed.), *Carmichael's manual of child psychology* (pp. 245–283). New York: Wiley.

Prutting, C. A. (1979). The process: The action of moving forward progressively from one point to another on the way to completion. *Journal of Speech and Hearing Disorders, 44,* 3–30.

Ratusnik, D. L., and Koenigsknecht, R. A. (1975). Influence of certain clinical variables on Black preschoolers' nonstandard phonological and grammatical performance. *Journal of Communication Disorders, 8,* 281–297.

Seymour, H. N., and Miller-Jones, D. (1981). Language and cognitive assessment of Black children. In N. Lass (Ed.), *Speech and language: advances in basic research and practise* (Vol. 6). New York: Academic Press.

Seymour, H. N., and Seymour, C. M. (1977). A therapeutic model for communicative disorders among children who speak Black English vernacular. *Journal of Speech and Hearing Disorders, 42,* 247–256.

Seymour, H. N., and Seymour, C. M. (1981). Black English and standard American English contrasts in consonantal development for four- and five-year-old children. *Journal of Speech and Hearing Disorders, 46,* 276–280.

Slobin, D. I. (1979). *Psycholinguistics* (2nd ed.). Palo Alto, CA: Scott, Foresman and Company.

Sinclair-DeZwart, H. (1969). Developmental psycholinguistics. In D. Elkind and J. Flavell (Eds.), *Studies in cognitive development.* New York: Oxford University Press.

Stockman, I. J., and Vaughn-Cooke, F. B. (1981). *Semantic categories in the language of working class Black children.* Paper presented at Second International Child Language Conference, Vancouver, B.C.

Toliver-Weddington, G. (Ed.). (1979). Ebonics (Black English): Implications for education. *Journal of Black Studies, 9,* 364–366.

Vaughn-Cooke, F. B. (1983). Improving language assessment in minority children. *ASHA, 25,* 29–34.

Wolfram, W., and Fasold, R. W. (1974). *The study of social dialects in American English.* Englewood Cliffs, NJ: Prentice-Hall.

Wolfram, W. (1983). Test interpretation and sociolinguistic differences. *Topics in Language Disorders, 3,* 21–34.

Chapter 6

Clinical Intervention for Language Disorders Among Nonstandard Speakers of English

Harry N. Seymour

In treating language disorders, the clinician has two major responsibilities: (1) the establishment of interventional goals, and (2) the implementation of intervention goals. The six principles described in Chapter 5 are important to the effectiveness with which these responsibilities are carried out when working with nonstandard English speaking children. With this in mind, the following discussion proposes strategies, based on the six principles, for the establishment and implementation of intervention goals.

ESTABLISHMENT OF INTERVENTION GOALS

The establishment of intervention goals requires the formulation of hypotheses about a child's language competencies (Bloom and Lahey, 1978). This task is particularly difficult when working with the nonstandard English speaker because the clinician is often unable to differentiate nonstandard linguistic features from features that are symptomatic of language learning problems (Seymour and Seymour, 1977; Taylor, 1980). The source of this difficulty is twofold. First, clinicians are often unclear about the distinctions among the symptoms of language disorders, the causes of these disorders, and the features of nonstandard English. Second, there is an inadequate data base on language acquisition among nonstandard English speakers. The following discussion elaborates on these two problems and suggests possible solutions.

Causes and Symptoms of Disorders and Nonstandard English

Nonstandard English is neither a cause nor a symptom of language disorders. Language disorders typically are neurological, sensory, psychoemotional, and cognitive-intellectual in nature. The symptoms of these deficits, when grouped according to syndromes, form categories that are labeled learning disabilities, hearing impairment, autism, and mental retardation. How these pathological categories affect language functioning is little influenced by a speaker's dialect. The symptoms of language impairment reduce the capacity of both standard and nonstandard English speakers to communicate effectively. Deficiencies in the production or comprehension of language may be characterized by difficulties with word finding, semantic organization, pragmatics, mathetics, syntax, morphemes, and phonemes, among others; these difficulties should not be confused with features of nonstandard English.

Yet, because certain features of nonstandard English are similar in form to some characteristics of language disorders, there is potential for confusion. It must be understood, however, that a disordered language system or profile is far more pervasive in deviant characteristics than the relatively limited number of features identified with particular nonstandard dialects. A case made for clinical intervention on behalf of a child who presents only those features that are associated with nonstandard English patterns would be a poor one. On the other hand, children with language disorders will show areas of deficit that go beyond the forms characterized by nonstandard dialectal patterns.

Limited Acquisitional Data

A second reason for clinicians' problems with separating symptoms of language disorders and nonstandard English patterns is the dearth of normative data on acquisition of language among nonstandard English speakers. A prevailing position is that many of the clinical problems surrounding nonstandard English would be resolved with greater knowledge of acquisitional milestones among nonstandard dialects (Cole, 1979; Vaughn-Cooke, 1983). Few can argue against this position. However, although normative data are certainly needed and would be helpful, they represent no panacea. We need only look at the standard English speaking child for whom there is considerable normative data to realize that these data are merely guidelines for clinical decisions.

In the discussion on the child-centered model (Chapter 5), it was pointed out that language development among standard English speakers is synergistic and highly variable. Developmental milestones are simply averages around which children can be quite different. Perhaps the most important developmental information for clinicians is the existence of general knowledge about what children tend to acquire and the general sequence of that acquisition. Table 6–2 shows a broad framework for acquisition. A general framework such as this can be helpful as a guide because variability between standard English and nonstandard English is most likely to occur within these stages rather than across them. Children are unlikely to acquire two word phrases before single words or complex sentences before inflectional modulations, for example. But they may differ in the acquisitional sequence of morphemic inflections, such as present progressive -*ing,* plural -*s,* possessive *'s,* and so forth (Crystal, Fletcher, and Garman, 1976; deVilliers and deVilliers, 1973).

Indeed, there is no evidence that children of nonstandard English backgrounds would perform differently relative to these broad five stages. Black English speaking children begin with one word semantic relations, progress to modulations in meaning, then to sentence modulations, and so forth. Of course, Brown's five stages are based on mean length of utterance (MLU), which should not be applied to nonstandard English speaking children because of the absence of norms and the standard English bias associated with counting inflectional morphemes. Despite this difference, the progression from Stage I to Stage V appears predictable for all children acquiring the English language (Brown, 1973; Slobin, 1979).

However, as with the standard English-speaking child, there will be variations within stages and, of course, certain nonstandard English features will alter the structural profile within these stages. For instance, many children in the sentence modulation stage will omit morphemic inflections, but others will not. Or, because of code switching, children will use certain nonstandard forms in some contexts and not in others. Hence, there is considerable opportunity for variability among nonstandard English speakers. For this reason, normative developmental profiles can serve as only rough guides in establishing intervention goals.

An alternative approach to exclusive reliance on normative developmental profiles is to have a child-centered and bidialectal focus.

Table 6–1. Brown's Five Stages of Sentence Construction

Stage I	*Relations or roles within the simple sentence* Content: Semantic and relational functions
Stage II	*Modulations of meaning within the simple sentence* Content: Acquisition of grammatical morphemes
Stage III	*Modalities of the simple sentence* Content: Acquisition of question, negation, and imperative transformations
Stage IV	*Embedding of one sentence within another* Content: Acquisition of embedding of object-noun comple- ment, wh-question, and relative clause
Stage V	*Coordination of simple sentence and propositional relations* Content: Acquisition of complex sentences

Adapted from Brown, R. (1973). *A first language.* Cambridge, MA: Harvard University Press.

Instead of using psychometric normative data of standardized tests for determining a child's language competencies, a single-subject approach is taken. This single-subject approach determines a child's productive language capacity by sampling and probing language behavior. A discussion of productive capacity, language sampling, and the language probing process follows.

Productive Capacity

An important aspect of this alternative approach is the determination of the extent to which forms are a productive part of the child's language system. Productive capacity is defined here as evidence of consistent production of a language pattern. A consistent pattern may be either standard or nonstandard. However, because nonstandard forms may not be differentiated easily from pathological forms when working with language disordered children, it is more practical to focus initially on patterns that do not vary from standard forms.

Evidence of consistent patterns derives from the percentage of occurrence of forms in obligatory contexts. Thus, production ratios for the number of times concepts are coded by standard English forms provide an important profile of the child's system. With such a profile, the clinician can focus attention on patterns that vary from standard English to differentiate those patterns from pathological behavior. This differentiation indicates the areas in which the child is having difficulties as well as his or her areas of strength. Information about language strengths and weaknesses for a child who has been identified as language disordered reflects the manner in which that child's language is unfolding. The direction for the clinician, then, is to plan intervention according to the child's emerging system by capitalizing on the strengths and eliminating the weaknesses. Such a child-centered approach minimizes a clinician's reliance on developmental normative data. The child's emerging system, although faulty, provides the guide for determining which language areas require attention.

A major question about nonstandard English speakers regarding this issue of productive capacity is how to interpret low percentage of occurrence for particular forms. If a child codes possession with the -s marker 20 percent of the time, codes action with the three major sentence components (subject, verb, and object) 40 percent of the time, and produces *on* preposition in a locative content category 70 percent of the time, that child would be regarded has having high productive capacity for the latter form but not the first two. What does this mean clinically?

It simply means that baseline measures of how the child is performing have been established. Designating that the child has low productive capacity need not imply that these forms are areas of weakness because they may be features of nonstandard English, not indicative of pathology. However, knowledge of productive capacity for language forms establishes baseline measures for further determination of whether patterns are weaknesses or strengths. Such a determination can most effectively be accomplished only through a thorough sampling and an in-depth analysis of language.

Language Sampling

The analysis of language should include a contrastive linguistic analysis between standard and nonstandard English features. However, a clinician should not rely solely on this kind of analysis for establishing goals. Because a contrastive analysis between dialects typically focuses on form and not on content or use (Seymour and Miller-Jones, 1981; Seymour and Seymour, 1977, 1981), there is too much information left out of the analysis. Although a child may delete morphological inflections for reasons of dialectal influences, these deletions may also occur because of a pathological condition. Lack of clarity on the distinction between symptoms of pathology and nonstandard English features makes identification of pathology difficult and treatment next to impossible. Hence, a more complete language profile is necessary.

A language profile provides necessary information for determining the direction for language facilitation. This profile will reflect standard and nonstandard English forms. The exact mix and combination can be assessed only by an analysis of the child's system. It is the in-depth analysis of subjects' language sample that provides *patterns* of behavior. These patterns are windows into a child's language system and are therefore answers to questions about language competency. How do children use transformations in the formation of questions, negations, conjunctions, and so forth? Is there evidence of embedding? Does this evidence encompass object-noun-complement, wh-clauses, and relative clauses, and, if it does, to what extent? And, perhaps as important as production measures, what does the child comprehend about these language forms?

Answers to these and other clinical questions are best obtained through language sampling. Although many clinicians attempt to determine the nature of a child's problem through standardized testing, there are many reasons for avoiding this approach with nonstandard English speakers (see Seymour and Miller-Jones, 1981; Taylor and Payne, 1983; and Vaughn-Cooke, 1983, for a detailed discussion of this issue). Indeed, the single strongest argument for the language sampling context, as opposed to standardized testing, is that it provides the opportunity to assess the child in a relatively naturalistic milieu. Stockman and Vaughn-Cooke (1981) and Seymour and Miller-Jones (1981) make a particularly strong and convincing argument that naturalistic language sampling overcomes the constraints and limitations associated with highly structured elicitation formats, such as standardized tests of language, sentence repetition tasks, cloze procedures, sentence completion tasks, and so forth.

The closer the assessment process is to a naturalistic communicative interaction between clinician and child, the more likely the language produced by the child will be generative and reflect an interaction among dimensions. Given a multidimensional, interactive, and generative product, the clinician can evaluate co-occurring dynamics among form-content-use and the child's capacity to generate forms appropriate to linguistic and nonlinguistic contexts. With this information, hypotheses may be formulated about the nature of the language problem.

Language Probing Process

Once a clinician has formulated hypotheses about a child's language these hypotheses must be tested. This author proposes that the testing of the hypotheses be accomplished through a language probing process (LPP). The concept of language probes is not new, and their use has been proposed for children of nonstandard English backgrounds (Leonard and Weiss, 1983). The LPP discussed in this chapter is similar to criterion referenced assessment in that it involves determining the behavior or domain of language to be assessed and conducting an in-depth probe of that domain (Glaser and Nitko, 1971). Although not commonly used in the field of communication disorders, criterion referenced assessment offers considerable promise. Unlike norm referenced testing, criterion referenced tests focus on the domain of information that the individual being tested is supposed to know (Gorth and Hambleton, 1972). There are no group comparisons made relative to distributional rankings. The examiner is more interested in information about what the child knows as opposed to how that child compares to other children of his or her peer group. Hence, an individual child's performance on a criterion referenced test indicates how well that child has mastered a particular competency area.

Although the general purpose is similar, the LPP differs from traditional criterion referenced assessment tests. First and foremost, LPP is not a test but an assessment process. As such, there is no test standardization and the assessment is not a discrete stage but continues into the intervention phase of therapy (diagnostic-intervention). A second important difference is that with criterion referenced assessment tests data are interpreted in a criterion referenced manner. This means that there is a criterion, based on normative data, that establishes the level required for the mastery of a particular domain. Thus, in criterion referenced testing a criterion has been established prior to testing that determines mastery level for a domain of information. A good example of a criterion referenced interpretation of data is a 90 percent criterion for mastery of obligatory forms in standard English. Normative data suggest that mastery of standard English forms is strongly evident at a 90 percent performance level (Bloom and Lahey, 1978; Brown, 1973).

Contrastingly, an absolute criterion for mastery, such as 90 percent, applied to nonstandard English speakers could be biased, arbitrary, and inconsequential. This is particularly so for nonstandard English patterns because of the potential for variability in subject responses and the limited normative data on nonstandard English. Therefore, the clinician should be cautious about establishing a priori achievement criteria. A more practical approach, as earlier discussed under productive capacity, is to establish a profile of the child's production ratios on various tasks and interpret that profile relative to hypotheses being tested.

As an example of this process, assume for a hypothetical case that test results reveal a production ratio of 30 percent for present progressive -*ing* among various LPP tasks. In addition these findings fail to support an initial hypothesis that this child has productive capacity for the present progressive -*ing*. A performance of 30 percent, then, represents a baseline measure to be interpreted relative to the child's dialect and general developmental level. The implications concerning whether the production of -*ing* would be an intervention goal depend on the child's overall performance in terms of strengths and weaknesses for production or comprehension tasks for -*ing*, as well as on other measures.

Herein lies the major advantage of LPP, in that the assessment process can reveal the client's strengths and weaknesses. The major difficulty with norm referenced tests is that they test too few items within a domain to be validly representative of the domain. As a consequence, a norm referenced test of language allows a clinician to determine how well a child does on the test in comparison to other children but yields insufficient information about the child's strengths and weaknesses. This problem is remedied with the LPP.

In Table 6–2 there is a demonstration of a sequence of activities that represent an attempt to assess the hypothesis that a child has productive capacity for -*s* morphemic inflections in possessive, plural, and third person subject-verb agreement. This sequence of activities, adapted from intervention formats proposed by Wiig and Semel (1980), illustrates how a clinician can probe a particular domain to assess a child's competency within that domain. The suggested activities are examples only and would be expanded in an actual clinical context. There are many tasks typically used in assessment and intervention that may be adapted for purposes of probing a domain of language. The challenge before the clinician is to select tasks that provide the kinds of data necessary for understanding the child's language strengths and weaknesses.

There are three aspects of LPP exemplified in Table 6–2 that are considered essential. First, there should be numerous tasks that assess the same function and a variety of items within each task. Variety is important because the object of the assessment is to elicit sufficient information to discern a *pattern* of behavior that is indicative of underlying knowledge about the domain being tested. Moreover, when a variety of items and activities are used, the likelihood of assessing the targeted domain is greater, and therefore the assessment process becomes more valid. Also, the confounding effects of idiosyncratic responses are reduced by presenting several items.

The second consideration in LPP is to diversity the linguistic and, if possible, nonlinguistic environments. The purpose here is to determine the extent to which linguistic and nonlinguistic constraints affect the use of specific language forms. Information of this kind can be useful in determining the child's knowledge about a par-

Table 6–2. Language Probing Process (LPP) of -s Morphemic Inflection

	RESPONSE
STIMULI	*(right/wrong)

Task 1: Recognition and Judgment of Correct Form

1. The boys *walk* to school.
2. There are two *book*.
3. That is *John* hat.
4. The girl *skips* rope.
5. I have one *toys*.
6. Give me *Harry's* shoe.

Task 2: Cloze Procedure   *Choose one:*

1. Mary _____ fast.   run/runs
2. I have many _____.   apple/apples
3. _____ cake is delicious. Mother/Mother's
4. The men _____ hard.   work/works
5. He has fifty _____.   cent/cents
6. He stepped on _____ foot. Bill/Bill's

Task 3: Imitation   *Sentence repetition*

1. He writes with David's pencil.
2. Mike's horses run faster than Hank's dogs.
3. Luke goes fishing at two ponds.
4. *Her cats* scratch each other's ears.
5. Father breaks cups and saucers when doing dishes.

Task 4: Deep Structure Meaning   *Answer in complete sentences*

1. John is Pollys son who likes to fish and Sally is Polly's daughter who likes to swim.

Who are John and Sally? What does John like to do? What does Sally like to do?

2. The girls have three baseball bats and the boys have one baseball.

What do the girls have? How many balls are there?

3. Billy plays basketball and runs track.

What does Billy do?

*The clinician merely interprets the client's judgments without imposing a "correct" or "incorrect" response model.

ticular form and how best to present stimulus tasks in further assessment and intervention.

The third dimension depicted in this sequence of activities pertains to the interaction between production and comprehension. In testing nonstandard English speakers, it is of major importance to assess both comprehension and production. Without evidence of the child's understanding, many utterances under production tasks can be ambiguous to the clinician. The deletion of past tense *-ed*, for example, may mean the child is using a nonstandard English pattern, or this deletion could mean that the child has a language deficit, preventing production of the standard English form.

One way to examine the source of a deletion pattern is to assess the child's understanding of the concept of past tense. A child who fails to produce but still understands a form when heard in context is very different from the child who neither produces nor understands a particular form. In this regard, nonstandard English speaking children understand standard English forms even though they may not produce them. Although it is also possible for the language disordered child to exhibit production deficits for forms he or she understands in context, the process of probing through a combination of comprehension and production can lead to greater insight about the child's dialect and the nature of his or her problem.

The LPP makes it possible for the clinician to test hypotheses formulated from the analysis of the language sample. This process is also useful in revising hypotheses in response to a client's progress or lack thereof. By retesting the client on the same or similar language probing tasks, the clinician can determine whether and the manner in which intervention goals should be revised. Hence, LPP constitutes an ongoing evaluation of the efficacy of goals and of procedures for implementing those goals.

IMPLEMENTATION OF GOALS

The foregoing discussion provided the rationale for the selection of intervention goals. In this section a proposal shall be made as to how intervention goals might be implemented. Two factors directly influence the implementation of goals: (1) the cause of the language impairment, and (2) the methods available for altering language behavior. These factors are discussed in the following paragraphs.

Etiology

Until now the emphasis in establishing goals has been on language symptoms, not on the various causes behind those symptoms. A current view is that knowledge about causes and categorical labels for language disorders are of less importance in establishing intervention goals than in implementation of these goals (Bloom and

Lahey, 1978; Muma, 1978). Advocates of this position assert that the underlying causes of language disorders, unlike language symptoms, often are not amenable to clinical intervention. Indeed, the clinician can do very little in altering precipitating causes of language disorders, such as cognitive-intellectual and neurological deficits. However, the capacity of the child to function linguistically within the limitations imposed by the deficit can be improved through intervention.

Still another reason for emphasizing language symptoms over causes in the establishment of goals is that little information about the nature of the language problem may be gained by knowing either the category of disability or its cause. Children who fall within such categories as mental retardation, learning disability, hearing impairment, and autism are very different. These categories do not constitute homogeneous groupings with respect to language symptoms, personality, intelligence, and so forth. Hence, knowing the category can only result in gross predictions about the nature of the language symptoms. Therefore, the same routine in analyzing a child's language profile is recommended regardless of causation.

The importance of etiology comes into focus when goals are to be implemented. Although children with disorders of different causes or categorical syndromes may have similar intervention goals, the approach to carrying out those goals will be affected by the child's handicapping condition. A child who is hearing impaired and of normal intelligence will be approached differently from a child who is mentally retarded. A very attentive language delayed child will require less structure than an autistic child who is hyperactive. Thus, the cause of the disorder influences the selection of methods of intervention and the possible structural framework in which goals are to be implemented, but not what those goals are to be. This is true for the nonstandard English speaking child as well as the standard English speaking child.

Methods

The selection of methods used to implement intervention goals is influenced by both pathological language symptoms and causation. Their selection should be in accordance with the potential for eliminating or reducing pathology and for suitability relative to the physical or psychological limitations of the child. Although the factor of nonstandard English is an overriding concern throughout the intervention process from initial assessment to intervention methods, it is the child's individual needs (child-centered approach) that ultimately determine what the methods shall be.

Regarding the child's individual needs, it must be kept in kind that deficits affect children's learning of language differently. In fact, no two children speaking even the same dialect will likely have the same set of linguistic features resulting from a particular cause. Aside from dialectal differences, symptoms associated with language disorders will vary among children because their learning environment and physiological and psychological makeups are different. The features of dialect are incidental to the potential myriad of pathological language symptoms. The challenge for the clinician is to specify as clearly as possible the nature of the child's language problem and to implement intervention strategies that make the child a more effective language learner.

The phrase "more effective language learner" does not imply that the child should necessarily be taught standard English, or, for that matter, any particular dialect. The child must acquire that which is common to all dialects — the ability to induce rules of language from the environment so that effective language may be generated. The particular dialect a child happens to speak depends on the social context in which the language learning process has taken place. It is the language learning process (the inducement of rules) that is fundamental, however, and should be the clinician's primary focus, rather than the specific dialect involved.

This language learning process is generative, multidimensional, interactional, and, in the case of the nonstandard English speaking child, bidialectal. Thus, methods selected for intervention must support a learning plan that encompasses these factors. To achieve such a learning plan, efforts should be made to implement goals within a language learning context that is as natural as possible; that provides the opportunity for the child to combine form, content, and use of language; that encourages bidialectal behavior; and that is individualized to meet the specific needs of the child.

The single most important obstacle to implementing a language learning plan of this kind is the extent to which a client can attend simultaneously to multiple stimuli. The factor of attention determines the degree of structure and the number of intervention goals that are possible. The clinician should impose the minimal level of structure at which the client can demonstrate success, and then progressively move the client toward more naturalistic and less structured contexts. For, the more unnatural the intervention format, the more artificial the communicative interaction between client and clinician and the less likely will the aforementioned clinical principles be followed.

Table 6–3 shows methods appropriate for highly structured contexts and Table 6–4 lists some methods considered appropriate for contexts that are low in structure. For each method, examples are provided that are suggestive of the kinds of tasks that can go on between clinician and client, but these examples are not meant to be exhaustive. The kinds of activities that can be selected are limited only by the imagination and skill of the clinician. However, the clinician should be guided by the single motive of making the child an independent language user, capable of generating language to express a wide range of communicative intents.

Among the highly structured methods there are *imitation, sentence completion, cloze procedures,* and *multiple choice tasks* (Table 6–3). These methods may be used singly or in combination in implementing intervention goals. They provide the opportunity to test both production and comprehension on the part of the child within a structured context. Of course, which methods and kinds of tasks within each method should be used depends on the child's language level. It is important to keep in mind that the child's own behavior relative to his or her language strengths and weaknesses provides the direction of the language plan.

In this regard, examples given in Table 6–3 reflect intervention goals that have standard English as target behaviors in addition to Black English target forms. In keeping with the bidalectal principle that nonstandard English speakers also comprehend and, to varying degrees, produce standard English, goals may reflect one or both dialects. The extent to which either dialect is used as target behavior depends on the individual child's linguistic repertoire as well as on his or her environmental home and school circumstances. Such decisions must be made on an individual basis and should not be determined by a priori sets of linguistic features considered standard or nonstandard. Instead, target forms of either dialect are used to strengthen the child's competency in understanding and producing language generally, not necessarily a specific dialect.

Moreover, the aim of the clinician is to establish, as soon as is possible, a low structured and naturalistic learning context for the child. In such a context there is maximum opportunity to work on many goals simultaneously and within an environment that simulates natural language use. It is widely held that children can best induce rules of language in situations that closely approximate how language is learned naturally (Berry, 1980; Bloom and Lahey, 1978;

Table 6-3. Language Intervention Methods for a Highly Structured Clinical Setting

Imitation
Purpose:
Client reproduces model provided by the clinician to establish auditory image of target form.

Example:
Clinician: "The man kick*ed* a football."
Client: "The man kick*ed* a football."

Sentence Completion
Purpose:
Client relies on clues from a partial sentence (stimuli) to recall and generate appropriate forms located at the end of the sentence.

Example:
Clinician: "This glass has more water."
          "This glass has _____ water."
          (Stimuli are glasses with different quantities of water.)
Client: "This glass has *less* water."

Cloze Procedure
Purpose:
The client generates an appropriate form omitted from the sentence stimulus. This differs from sentence completion in that the form may be omitted from anywhere in the sentence rather than just at the end.

Example:
Clinician: "Michael Jackson _____ a singer _____ a dancer."
Client: "Michael Jackson *is* a singer *and* a dancer."

Multiple Choice Task
Purpose:
Client focuses in on attributes of a form by selecting one among others that may be similar in meaning. This task may be used with sentence completion and cloze procedure.

Example:
Clinician: "The airplane fell to earth and _____."
Client: (fired, broked, *crashed*)

Lund and Duchan, 1983; Muma, 1978). Some methods illustrative of this kind of learning are *modeling, parallel talk,* and *communication games.*

Modeling may include several tactics. Among various versions, *correction, expansion,* and *alternation* are common clinical procedure. The child provides the stimulus in conversational discourse and the clinician responds by either correcting what has been said, expanding on the utterance, or providing an alternative to the utterance (Table 6-4). Correction alters a specific form, expansion provides a revised version that builds on the initial form, and alternation provides a different form that expresses the same function.

Table 6–4.   Language Intervention Methods for Low Structured Settings

Modeling
Purpose:
  Client is provided with an example of desired stimuli so that an appropriate auditory image may be formed.

Example (Correction):
  Client: "I no want it."
  Clinician: "I don't want it."

Example (Expansion):
  Client: "Me run."
  Clinician: "You run fast."

Example (Alternation):
  Client: "Mommy cook."
  Clinician: "Your mother is going to bake a cake."

Parallel Talk
Purpose:
  Client experiences an immediate model that amplifies his or her own utterance within the natural communicative context.

Example:
  Client: (Context: Child is playing with a truck)
              "tuck,"   "dive,"   "tuck go."
  Clinician: "tuck,"   "dive tuck,"   *"truck* go."

Communication Game
Barrier Game: A screen serves as a barrier separating the speaker (client) and the listener (clinician).

Example:
  Client describes to the clinician how to arrange colored blocks to form a house.

  Client: "First put red block on blue block. Next put green block. Then put blue block on orange block and put another red block on it. That's a house."
  Clinician: The clinician, as listener, attempts to follow the client's instructions. The results indicate how well the client has communicated his intentions.

Over-the-Shoulder Game: Repeat the foregoing actions, but without the barrier. The client observes listener progress and, as a result, is able to employ feedback and monitoring skills to modify his or her instructions.

Modeling methods are valuable clinical tools when working with nonstandard English speaking children. Mindful of the bidialectal language background of these children, the clinician might have to model alternative forms of "correctness." Indeed, the child has the option of articulating /θ/ or /f/——> [θ] in the final-word position of "mouth" or deleting -*ed* past tense marker in "play(ed)." Consequently, modeling of code switching on the part of the clinician can be carried off effectively by presenting contrastive forms among the correction, expansion, and alternation options.

Parallel talk is also a version of modeling, which involves "echoing" the client's utterances. However, parallel talk contrasts with the versions of modeling presented earlier in that the clinician's role is less intrusive and obvious. The clinician talks about what the child is discussing at a language level that parallels that of the child. It takes place during natural conversation and allows the clinician to emphasize and embellish aspects of the child's utterances that are consistent with intervention goals. No attempt is made to correct the child. An important aspect of parallel talk is the spontaneity of the child's utterance and the clinician's simultaneous embellishments. Muma (1978) points out four advantages of parallel talk: It mirrors the child's language level; it is timely; it includes the child's communicative intent; and it combines form and function.

In parallel talk, the child's conversation is the clinical focus. The clinician repeats pertinent elements of what the child has said and attempts to mold and shape aspects of language form and function within the natural conversational context. It is the child who generates the language stimuli spontaneously. This factor is particularly important with nonstandard English speaking children. Because there are often cultural, ethnic, and socioeconomic differences between the clinician and the child, the clinician has a tendency to impose conversational stimuli and topics that may not be culturally or topically salient for the child. If the child is allowed to select the topic and the manner in which the topic is to be discussed, the clinician then simply builds on what the child provides. Thus, the child is more interested, more motivated, and more responsive to the clinician's parallel talking, and there is greater opportunity for reinforcement and carryover.

Another method for low-structured intervention is the communication game, of which there are various versions. Two that are particularly useful for focusing on use of language are what Muma (1978) refers to as the "barrier game" and the "over-the-shoulder" game. The barrier game makes use of a barrier (screen) between speaker and listener. Stimulus items are duplicated on each side of the screen. The task is for the speaker (the client) to arrange the items in a particular way and to instruct the listener (clinician or another client) in duplicating that arrangement. The extent to which the listener is able to follow the instructions depends on the communicative effectiveness of the speaker.

A variation of this procedure is the over-the-shoulder game, which allows the speaker to observe the action of the listener in following the speaker's instructions. In this second task, the barrier has been removed and the speaker receives immediate feedback on how well he or she is instructing the listener. The speaker then responds to the listener's actions by modifying his or her instructions in accordance with the listener's needs. In addition to focusing on production aspects of language, the clinician has the opportunity to strengthen listening skills as well by changing the clinician-client roles.

The communication games develop speaker awareness of their effect on the listener. Certain pragmatic skills, such as listener presupposition, feedback, and monitoring, can be improved. These skills have particular implications for nonstandard English speakers because of the interpersonal dynamics of bidialectism. Nonstandard English speaking children often switch codes because of feedback received from the listener. This listener reaction may be positive or negative, depending upon the listener's attitude and the context. If the child perceives negative or hostile feedback, he or she may become reticent or communicatively inept. Thus, for the language disordered child it is important to learn about standard English and Black English contrasts and how an individual can effectively switch styles as listener and speaking contexts change. The communicative games can help make that happen.

SUMMARY

The methods proposed in this chapter are based on "state of the art" practices in language intervention but have been adapted for the nonstandard English speaking child. Although complex questions remain about the diagnosis and treatment of children of linguistically diverse backgrounds, there are reasons for optimism. As implied in this chapter, answers are likely to come from a greater understanding of the relationship between structure and function of language and from new advances made in nonstandardized and naturalistic diagnostic-intervention methods. Thus, current professional interest in these areas bodes well for the client of any dialectal background.

REFERENCES

Berry, M.F. (1980). *Teaching linguistically handicapped children.* Englewood Cliffs, NJ: Prentice-Hall.

Bloom, L., and Lahey, M. (1978). *Language development and language disorders.* New York: Wiley.

Brown, R. (1973). *A first language.* Cambridge, MA: Harvard University Press.

Cole, L. (1979). *Developmental analysis of social dialect features in the spontaneous language of preschool Black children.* Unpublished doctoral dissertation, Northwestern University, Chicago.

Crystal, D., Fletcher, P., and Garman, M. (1976). *The grammatical analysis of language disability.* New York: Elsevier.

deVilliers, J.G., and deVilliers, P.A. (1973). A cross-sectional study of the acquisition of grammatical morphemes in child speech. *Journal of Psycholinguistic Research, 2,* 267–278.

Glaser, R., and Nitko, A. (1971). Measurement in learning and instruction. In R. Thorndike (Ed.), *Educational measurement* (pp. 625–670). Washington, DC: American Council on Education.

Gorth, W., and Hambleton, R. (1972). Measurement considerations for criterion-referenced testing and special education. *Journal of Special Education, 6,* 303–314.

Leonard, L.B., and Weiss, A.L. (1983). Application of nonstandardized assessment procedures to diverse linguistic populations. *Topics in Language Disorders, 3*(3), 35–45.

Lund, J.N., and Duchan, J.F. (1983). *Assessing children's language in naturalistic contexts.* Englewood Cliffs, NJ: Prentice-Hall.

Muma, J. (1978). *Language handbook, concepts, assessment, intervention.* Englewood Cliffs, NJ: Prentice-Hall.

Seymour, H.N., and Miller-Jones, D. (1981). Language and cognitive assessment of Black children. In N. Lass (Ed.), *Speech and language: Advances in basic research and practise,* Vol. 6 (pp. 203–263). New York: Academic Press.

Seymour, H.N., and Seymour, C.M. (1977). A therapeutic model for communicative disorders among children who speak Black English vernacular. *Journal of Speech and Hearing Disorders, 42,* 247–256.

Seymour, H.N., and Seymour, C.M. (1981). Black English and standard American English contrasts in consonantal development for four- and five-year-old children. *Journal of Speech and Hearing Disorders, 46,* 276–280.

Slobin, D.I. (1979). *Psycholinguistics* (2nd Ed.). Palo Alto, CA: Scott, Foresman and Company.

Stockman, I.J., and Vaughn-Cooke, F.B. (1981). *Child language acquisition in Africa and the diaspora: A neglected linguistic issue.* Paper presented at The First World Congress on Black Communication, Nairobi, Kenya.

Taylor, O.L. (1980). Communication disorders in Blacks. In B.E. Williams and O.L. Taylor (Eds.), *International Conference on Black Communication* (pp. 62–89). New York: The Rockefeller Foundation.

Taylor, O.L., and Payne, K.T. (1983). Culturally valid testing: A proactive approach. *Topics in Language Disorders, 3*(3), 8–20.

Vaughn-Cooke, F.B. (1983). Improving language assessment in Minority children. *American Speech-Language-Hearing Association, 25,* 29–34.

Wiig, E.H., and Semel, E.M. (1980). *Language assessment and intervention for the learning disabled.* Columbus, OH: Charles E. Merrill.

Chapter 7

A Cultural and Communicative Approach to Teaching Standard English as a Second Dialect

Orlando L. Taylor

BACKGROUND

Much controversy exists on the role, if any, of the speech-language pathologist in teaching standard English to nonstandard English speakers. Prior to the early 1970s this issue was not an issue! That is, until then, the discipline of communication disorders tended to view nonstandard English dialects—and many foreign accents—as pathological linguistic systems that were to be "improved," if not eradicated, by the speech-language pathologist. In other words, there was no discussion of teaching standard English as a *second* dialect. It was solely a matter of teaching standard English as a first—and only—language.

In the 1970s, several events occurred that influenced the profession's perspectives and policies vis-à-vis nonstandard English dialects. First, a few special interest groups (e.g., the Black Caucus of the American Speech and Hearing Association) called for a reassessment of definitions and norms for viewing normalcy and disorders among nonstandard English speakers (see Taylor, Stroud, Hurst, Moore, and Williams, 1969). Second, the field of sociolinguistics provided strong theoretical arguments, historical facts, and research data to demonstrate that nonstandard English dialects were linguistically valid, useful to their speakers, and devoid of inherent pathology. Third, Public Law 94-142, the Education of All Handicapped Children Act of 1975, prohibited the use of discriminatory assessment instruments that were not in the language or communication system of the person being assessed. This prohibition provided, by implication, enormous credibility to nonstandard English dialects. Finally, several court cases, such as *Lau v. Nichols* (1974) and *Martin Luther King Junior Elementary School Children v. Ann Arbor School District* (1979), established that educational programs that do not take a child's indigenous language into account violate the child's equal protection under the law as guaranteed by the 14th amendment to the United States Constitution.

The net result of these events has been to heighten the recognition that there is a significant difference between a language *difference* and a language *disorder.* It has not been established, however, what, if anything, should be done about these differences, or what the role of the speech-language pathologist should be in the event that intervention is the response of choice.

In 1983, the American Speech-Language-Hearing Association (ASHA) moved to correct the ambiguity between definition and pedagogy. Through a formal position paper on social dialects,* ASHA reiterated its view that a language difference should not be equated with a language disorder. ASHA went beyond this, however, and took the position that it may be advantageous for nonstandard English speakers to be able to speak standard English. It also asserted that it was proper for the speech pathologist, on an elective basis, to teach standard English to nonstandard English speakers.

To be qualified to teach standard English as an elective clinical service, however, ASHA claimed that the speech-language pathologist must (1) be sensitive to and competent in the linguistic features of the learner's indigenous dialect; (2) understand the effects of negative language attitudes on language performance; and (3) be familiar with linguistic contrastive analysis procedures.

This writer disagrees with ASHA's position on two important points. First, the statement fails to state explicitly the desired status of the learner's nonstandard English dialect while standard English is being taught. In other words, is the nonstandard dialect to be eradicated and replaced with standard English, or is the dialect to be preserved as a linguistic system equal to standard English, each dialect being used according to the situational and audience demands of individual communicative events? A growing body of research (cf. Cummins, 1981) shows clearly that it is unnecessary—indeed socially and cognitively undesirable—for a child's first or

---

*ASHA's 1983 Position Paper on Social Dialects is reprinted in Appendix A.

Basic Interpersonal Communication System (BICS) to be either eradicated or denied opportunity for full development to teach another linguistic system, in this case standard English. This second system, which is usually the language of education, may be thought of as the Cognitive Academic Language System (CALS).

A second problem with ASHA's position on social dialects is that it considers the teaching of standard English as a *clinical* rather than an *educational* issue. Clinical issues involve matters of rehabilitation and treatment of communication disorders. Educational issues involve matters of teaching new information to learners. An educational, rather than a clinical, orientation does not presume the learner's indigenous communicative behavior to be pathological.

Generally speaking, it is the role of the classroom teacher—not of the speech-language pathologist—to teach standard English, either as a replacement dialect or a second dialect. Occasionally, the speech-language pathologist is asked to provide consultative services in this process.

This chapter is written from the following perspectives:

1. All varieties of English are linguistically valid, have merit, and are reflective of the cultural, cognitive, and social orientations of their speakers.
2. It is reasonable for a society to have a linguistic standard that permits communication, education, and commerce across various speech communities.
3. The *teaching* of standard English to nonstandard English speakers does not require eradication of the nonstandard English system. Therefore, the teaching of standard English to nonstandard English speakers should be culturally based to the extent that the learner is taught to be bidialectal—that is, capable of controlling the linguistic system of both the home culture and the larger society for use when needed. This approach is often referred to as a "Standard English as a Second Dialect (SESD)" approach.
4. The teaching of standard English as a first or as a second dialect is the responsibility of teachers, *not* clinicians.
5. The speech-language pathologist, if knowledgeable about SESD procedures, can and should provide consultative services to classroom teachers and can, if the situation permits, switch from clinician to teacher to teach standard English as a second dialect.

The remainder of this chapter will be devoted to principles and techniques for teaching standard English as a second dialect. These principles and techniques were developed by the author and were field tested and refined in three California school districts.

Traditional Approaches for Teaching Standard English to Nonstandard English Speakers: A Legacy of Failure

The teaching of standard English to all learners is an implicitly and explicitly stated goal of the American school. Yet the national performance of the American school in teaching Standard English to nonstandard English speakers is dismal. On almost every reported measure at the national or state level, children from nonstandard English speaking communities achieve lower competency levels in the language of education than children who come from standard English speaking communities. The result has been an overplacement of nonstandard English speaking children in special education classes, speech-language pathology clinical services, and compensatory education classes, and an underplacement of these children in classes for talented and gifted students.

Why have traditional methodologies for teaching standard English to nonstandard English speakers failed? This author argues that these methodologies have failed primarily because they have been (1) prescriptive, (2) corrective, and (3) excessively structure focused. Moreover, the teaching methodologies have not been culturally based, and they have made little use of indigenous, nonstandard dialects, probably because of linguistic naiveté or negative attitudes toward language variation.

As stated earlier, the failure of schools to take students' indigenous language into account in the instructional process has been ruled unconstitutional (cf. *Lau v. Nichols,* 1975, and *Martin Luther King Junior Elementary School Children et al. v. Ann Arbor Michigan School District Board).* The Ann Arbor case specifically cited teacher ignorance of issues related to language variation and negative teacher attitudes.

Whatever the reason, the fact is that the nation's schools have failed to teach standard English to a large percentage of nonstandard English speaking students — perhaps the majority — and this failure has contributed to the assessment and placement issues cited earlier. In addition, this failure has contributed to diminished student self-esteem, lowered teacher expectations, and discipline problems.

Developing Alternative Approaches to Teaching Standard English as a Second Dialect

If we are to develop an effective alternative to the traditional and failure-ridden approaches to teaching standard English as a second dialect, three prerequisite steps must be taken. First, the teacher dialect, three prerequisite steps must be taken. First, the teacher must eradicate any misconceptions that he or she might have pertaining to the nature of nonstandard English speech communities and to the pedagogical requirements for teaching any new linguistic system to a learner. Second, the teacher should become familiar with basic principles of second dialect instruction. Third, the teacher should become familiar with the guidelines developed by the Speech Communication Association and the American Speech-Language-Hearing Association (Standards for Effective Communications Programs, n.d.).

Some Common Myths About Language and Teaching New Linguistic Systems

It is not uncommon for teachers to approach the task of teaching standard English to nonstandard English speakers with a number of misconceptions about language differences. Teachers may also have misconceptions about how to teach a new linguistic system to a person who has a normal system developing or already in place. These misconceptions are usually outgrowths of general societal attitudes; a lack of formal training in linguistics, sociolinguistics, or second language instructional methods; or exposure to invalid research studies. Irrespective of their geneses, the SESD teacher must approach the task with as few of these misconceptions as possible.

In Table 7-1, a sample "Myth Assessment" instrument is presented. The reader is asked to indicate whether he or she agrees or disagrees with each statement. The appropriate answer for each item, based on available research, is presented at the bottom of Table 7-1. Presentation and discussion of myth assessment instruments, such as the one presented in Table 7-1, are a good way for SESD teachers to determine what they know — and don't know — about language, language variation, and teaching new linguistic systems. Subsequent readings in major text books in sociolinguistics (e.g., Fasold, 1984), ethnography of communication (e.g., Saville-Troike, 1982), and second language instruction are advisable. It is also advisable to consult articles written about language programs outside the United States that take into account indigenous language and dialects. Bamgbose's work in West Africa (1983), and Craig's work in Jamaica (1983), are excellent examples of such programs.

General Principles of Second Dialect Instruction

Having eliminated basic myths pertaining to language variation and the teaching of second linguistic systems, the clinician is now

Table 7-1. What Do I Know About Language?

Directions: Circle A for each of the following statements with which you agree or D for each statement with which you disagree.

A D   1. Standard English is the "correct" way to speak at all times.

A D   2. Standard English has more and better structure than other varieties of English.

A D   3. Southern English should not be considered a type of standard English.

A D   4. Standard English is white English.

A D   5. Poor people do not communicate as well as middle class people.

A D   6. Black people do not communicate as well as white people.

A D   7. Parents who do not speak standard English should talk little to their children to prevent them from developing bad speech habits.

A D   8. If a child is to learn standard English, he or she must "unlearn" any other variety of English that he or she speaks.

A D   9. Black American English is the same as southern English.

A D 10. Oral language instruction takes away from the time needed to teach children to read and write.

Answers: All items stated are common myths pertaining to language. Therefore, you should have disagreed with each item.

---

prepared to become familiar with some general principles of second dialect instruction.

Eleven of the basic principles are presented below:

1. The development of a positive attitude toward the existing dialect of the learner is a prerequisite for a second dialect instruc-

tional program. A positive attitude, however, is not an instructional program in and of itself.

2. Second dialect instruction is best taught to learners who want to learn another dialect. If motivation is not present, the teacher must facilitate the acquisition of that motivation by assisting the learner to discover advantages for acquiring the second dialect.

3. Both teacher and learner must believe that it is possible to acquire a second dialect.

4. Instruction in a second dialect must be preceded by a nonbiased assessment of the learner's knowledge of his or her first dialect and his or her knowledge of the targeted second dialect.

5. Selection of language and communication features to be taught in a second dialect instructional program should conform to language acquisition norms, stigmatization of first dialect features, frequency of occurrence of the features, and the learner's attitudes toward those features.

6. Second dialect instruction requires the teacher to know the linguistic and communicative rules of both the existing and the targeted dialect and the learner to be able to clearly recognize contrasts between the two.

7. Second dialect instruction must take into account cultural values associated with learning and teaching, including values pertaining to the roles of teachers and learners; various types of communicative behaviors; and the communicative teaching-learning environment.

8. Second dialect instruction must take into account the learning styles and preferences of the learners, including preferences pertaining to grouping configurations, social environment, level and type of competition, affective relationships with the teacher and other learners, and level of abstractness of materials.

9. Second dialect instruction must take into account the language goals and aspirations of the learner, his or her family, and his or her community.

10. Second dialect instruction is most effective when explicit linguistic and communicative features of the existing dialect are compared with those of the targeted dialect.

11. Second dialect instruction is best taught, especially to learners whose cultural orientations are non-Western, when instruction in language and communication is integrated with all aspects of the living culture of the learner.

These 11 principles probably do not exhaust the total number that should undergird SESD instruction. However, if they are consistently employed in instruction, the teacher has a greater likelihood of success than if they are ignored.

Guidelines for Oral Language Programs

In the final analysis, formal instruction in teaching Standard English as a second dialect is designed to improve an individual's competence in using a specific set of oral language skills to communicate specific intentions effectively in specific settings, to specific audiences, and on specific occasions. It would be useful, therefore, for the SESD teacher to become familiar with guidelines for implementing any type of oral communication program.

The most thorough set of guidelines for implementing oral communication programs was published in the late 1970s by a joint committee of the American Speech-Language-Hearing Association (ASHA) and the Speech Communication Association (SCA). These guidelines are presented in Appendix B.

The ASHA-SCA Standards for Effective Communication Programs will provide the reader with a detailed list of the following:

1. Basic definitions of the speaking *and* listening components of the communication process
2. Basic assumptions pertaining to communication competence and to oral communication instruction
3. The teaching and learning characteristics of effective oral communication program, with special emphases on (a) integration into the total academic curriculum, and (b) the pragmatic, situational, and stylistic aspects of instruction
4. The characteristics of support systems needed to facilitate effective instruction in such areas as personnel, parent or community involvement, and instructional resources
5. The characteristics of effective student assessments and program evaluations

ACCPT: A CULTURAL AND COMMUNICATIVE PROGRAM FOR TEACHING STANDARD ENGLISH AS A SECOND DIALECT

Only a few organized approaches are described in the literature for teaching standard English as a second dialect that take the first dialect of the learners into account and make no attempt to eradicate it. Most are built on principles established in bilingual education (cf. Feigenbaum, 1970). The three programs focus on the teaching of specific surface structure features of Standard English by means of (1) contrastive analysis procedures; (2) a variety of presentation, identification, translation, and response drills; and (3) an eventual focus on expansion activities into connected, spontaneous speech. Two excellent examples of the bilingual approach to second dialect instruction may be found in the programs designed to teach standard English as a second dialect in the school systems of Miami, Florida, and Oakland, California. A sample lesson plan from each of the Oakland Standard English Program (1984) is appended (see Appendix D). Note that the focus in the lesson is on the instruction of a specific morphological feature of standard English that differs from a morphological rule of Black English vernacular.

Although attractive in many aspects, the bilingual approach to teaching SESD tends to overemphasize the *structural* (linguistic) as opposed to the functional (communicative) aspect of instruction. As a result, its critics claim that the learner runs the risk of acquiring great competence in controlling the surface structure features of standard English, without necessarily knowing how to *use* these features—with the appropriate nonverbal and stylistic devices—to accomplish desired communicative intentions of their messages.

The approach to teaching SESD described on the next several pages attempts to link structural and communicative approaches to instruction. This approach has been developed by the author and is currently being field tested in a school system in the Western United States.

Like the bilingual oriented programs described above, this communicative approach to teaching SESD varies from traditional language education programs for nonstandard English speakers in that it does not "blame the victim." Moreover, it recognizes that the learning of standard English does not require denigration or elimination of students' indigenous language systems. Indeed, the program recognizes that the selection of language codes is situationally based and, for this reason, students need to retain their home language and dialects for use in the situations in which their use is appropriate. The program is orally based because of the recognition that oral language is the foundation for all language acquisition and learning, and that variations in oral language can—and typically do—influence the acquisition of competence in writing and reading standard English. Finally, the program is designed in such a way that it permeates the entire academic curriculum, not merely the language arts.

There are six basic tenets to the theoretical underpinnings for what may be called *A Cultural and Communication Program for Teaching Standard English as a Second Dialect* (ACCPTSESD or ACCPT—pronounced "accept"—for short). These tenets are as follows:

1. An oral focus
2. A "communicative" rather than a "structural" base
3. A three part focus: form, content, use
4. A linkage to "products"
5. A linkage across the curriculum
6. A linkage to a development teaching model

Each of these tenets is discussed further in the following paragraphs.

An Oral Focus

ACCPT is built around the premise that oral language is the primary vehicle for human communication. Oral language is universal in all cultures. Excluding exceptional cases, children acquire the oral language system of their culture with notable speed and ease and in an apparently universal manner. In short, oral language acquisition precedes all other forms of language acquisition, such as reading and writing, in most individuals and at all grade levels.

Oral language is at the heart of the language arts program in most school curricula, particularly in the elementary grades. Therefore, success in all aspects of language arts depends on the development and extension of the skills of oral language. For these reasons, every classroom during the developmental years should provide numerous opportunities for oral language practice, in some dialect, through activities, discussions, reports, and question and answer sessions.

A Communicative Focus

Traditionally, language arts programs have focused almost exclusively on the teaching of standard English structures, with little recognition given to the fact that effective communication requires more than mere *knowledge* of the linguistic features of a specific language system. Effective communication within any language system requires, in addition to knowledge of structural rules, knowledge of (1) the rules of conversations (e.g., turn taking, interruptions, etc., (2) rules for stringing sentences together in monologues and dialogues, (3) audience expectations for achieving the *functions* of communication (e.g., informing, controlling, imagining, stating feelings, ritualizing) and (4) nonverbal rules that accompany conversations.

ACCPT is built around the communicative aspects of human interaction, rather than around the relatively limited structural focus. Because structures are an integral part of communication, there is a place within the program for a focus on a specific linguistic structures in both listening and production activities.

A Three Part Focus

In any communication oriented instructional program, there should be three major foci: linguistic structure, communicative function, and underlying thought. Any one of these foci may be emphasize at one time, or various combinations may be emphasized, to heighten student competence in each. In any case, however, all three are always present in some form.

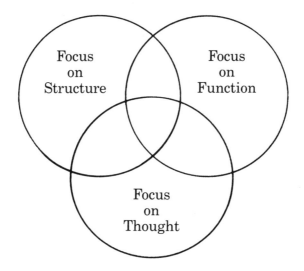

Focus on Structure

The focus on structure emphasizes use of the phonological, semantic, and grammatical rules considered to be appropriate for communicating specific intentions within a specific dialect.

When focusing on structure, lessons should combine direct instruction within a specific dialect, say standard English, with the student being provided with an abundance of opportunities to hear and practice the production of the targeted linguistic structures. It is essential that a real or imaginary audience and situation be defined within each lesson so that "correct" patterns do not become arbitrary but instead are directly related to the requirements of effective communication within a particular setting and before a specific audience.

Moreover, students should be given opportunities to listen to, contrast, and practice patterns of standard English with their indigenous dialect through lessons that address specific phonetic, lexical, or grammatical features. These opportunities should include discussions of similarities and differences among various dialects of English (including standard English as a set of socially acceptable language rules among those with political, economic, or educational power). They should be provided with opportunities to use the targeted structures in a variety of communication activities, such as choral reading, listening to various forms of literature, conversations and discussions with standard English speakers, Readers' Theater, and other dramatic activities.

Students in the upper grades might learn technical labeling of various features of standard English and other dialects. In the lower grades, however, an awareness of differences and the mastery of a variety of patterns would be the emphasis of instruction.

The focus on structure is an excellent place into which the bilingual oriented approaches discussed earlier can be integrated into ACCPT.

Focus on Function

Effective oral communication requires speakers to take into account the intent of their messages for various audiences and purposes. Students should learn to focus on what they are attempting to accomplish within a specific set of utterances and on the specific communicative and linguistic expectations of the audience. In other words, student should be able to determine the type of communicative behavior that would be most appropriate in a given situation and before a specific audience. For example, they might practice giving a message or presenting a persuasive argument on the same topic to various audiences—a classmate on the playground, the teacher in the classroom, or the school principal in her office. Each situation may require a different form of communication—for example, standard English (formal language) with the teacher or principal and the indigenous nonstandard English dialect (informal language) with the classmate. Students should be given an opportunity to decide, prior to a given activity, the type of communicative behaviors that would be most appropriate. Role playing of commonly encountered situations can help students use their understandings of daily life situations and relate these situations to the language forms most commonly acceptable for each.

Focus on Thought

Lessons that focus on thought address the underlying cognitive elements of language and communication. Here the focus is on such items as what the speaker is trying to tell the audience or the audience's interpretation of what has been heard and its communicative intention. To the extent that thinking involves language, research suggests that thought typically occurs in the person's primary language or dialect (BICS), the one he or she brings to school (Cummins, 1981).

Over time, however, the "thinking dialect" may change from the one associated with the BICS to the dialect associated with the CALS. Buckley (1976) claims that activities that enhance the students' language learning cannot take place in the traditional situation in which the teacher talks and the children are quiet. Instead, classroom activities should provide maximum opportunities for children to communicate with each other as partners or in small groups. New language learning is also thought to be facilitated by less emphasis on direct instruction and greater emphasis on facilitation of student interaction by such devices as questioning (i.e., open ended and thought provoking questions), and knowledge and experience sharing.

Finally, the atmosphere of the second dialect classroom must be positive. Instead of the traditional emphasis on "right" and "wrong" responses, the emphasis must be on making the learing environment one in which there is acceptance of differences among people, and where it is safe to risk being wrong, safe to evaluate one's own performance, and safe to try new ways of dealing with various situations. In such an environment, there is no "poor English" and no pattern of language is considered intrinsically "right" or intrinsically "wrong."

Finally, the focus on thought attempts to facilitate students' expansion of their fund of information through the integration of their own ideas with those from literature, the media, and other persons. It also is designed to teach students how to organize their ideas in such a way as to make them more effective in communicating their intentions.

Products

Teaching a language skill as an isolated phenomenon has been shown to be an ineffective strategy. Thus, the ACCPT concept argues that each lesson should be linked to short and long range "products," that is, to a specific set of tangible purposes and situations for which the particular skill being taught can be used (e.g., interviews, plays, dialogues, field trips, puppet shows, interpretative readings, and preparations for writing activities). In these various activities, students would be provided with tangible goals and directed purposes for using what they learn in drills and practice sessions. Without the designation of products, little carry-over is likely in SESD programs.

SESD Across the Curriculum

No type of oral language instruction, including SESD instruction, should be limited to the language instruction classroom. Therefore, effective SESD programs should make every effort to integrate SESD instruction with instruction in other academic areas. In this way, students will be able to see how competence in standard English relates to other subject areas, as well as how it might heighten their success in them. For example, in mathematics, students can be shown how knowledge in standard English can provide the essential link between mathematical concepts and their representation in numbers and in world problems.

In social studies, students may be given opportunities to organize material from various sources and translate it from written form to oral reporting. They might practice providing the same information in history, for example, to imaginary audiences in both the home (nonstandard) and school (standard) dialects. In this way, students have an opportunity to decide what they want to communicate and how they will tailor their presentations to meet the needs of their audience. They can also be given opportunities to practice the skills of classifying information and developing vocabulary to describe the various categories that they have used for organizing data.

The Developmental Sequence of Communication Teaching

In addition to the aforementioned three part focus, SESD instruction is more effective when it is conducted within a developmental framework. A developmental model has been developed for ACCPT that recognizes that acquisition of new or second dialect is not an all-or-none phenomenon. Instead, acquisition is more likely to proceed through an orderly process from the initial introduction of a particular aspect of language through its mastery. The ACCPT developmental model has been used to develop the aforementioned SESD programs in several school districts around the United States. The model is presented in Figure 7–1.

The model shown in Figure 7–1 is developmental in two ways. First, it schematizes the steps through which the learner must proceed when learning new forms of communication — a second dialect in this case — while preserving indigenous communicative systems for use in appropriate situations and on appropriate tasks. Second, it reflects the stages of growth that can permit an individual to go beyond a narrow, immediate, and inflexible view of language use to a broader, more flexible view.

Step I, *positive attitude toward own language,* is the foundation for all that is to come. It presumes that a fundamental prerequisite for second dialect learning is a respect for one's own language, as well as for the language of others. As we have stated so many times in this book, no dialect is intrinsically good or bad, correct or incorrect. All varieties of a language are tools for communicating ideas from person to person within a given speech community, depending on situation, topic, audience, and intention. The historical interaction between the powerful and the powerless in most societies has usually resulted in negative evaluation of the language of the powerless, a value loading that helps to perpetuate elitism and ethnocentrism. The primary, and continuing, job of the SESD teacher is to counteract this system of evaluation. Both learner *and* teacher must appreciate the various forms a specific language might take. This appreciation is facilitated by a deeper understanding of language in general, language standards, and the learner's indigenous language and communication systems.

The SESD classroom must reflect a positive atmosphere of respectful listening and enjoyment of the varieties of language that are heard. For older children, lessons might be developed on the historical evolution of various languages and dialects, regional differences, and similarities and differences among various language systems. From a developmental perspective, students should move from an emotional acceptance of the value of all languages, beginning with their own language, to an intellectual appreciation of language diversity. Thus, Step I is both primary and ongoing.

Step II involves *awareness of language varieties.* The young SESD learner, like most young children, is most likely to experience and analyze his or her world in relatively simple terms. The teacher's job

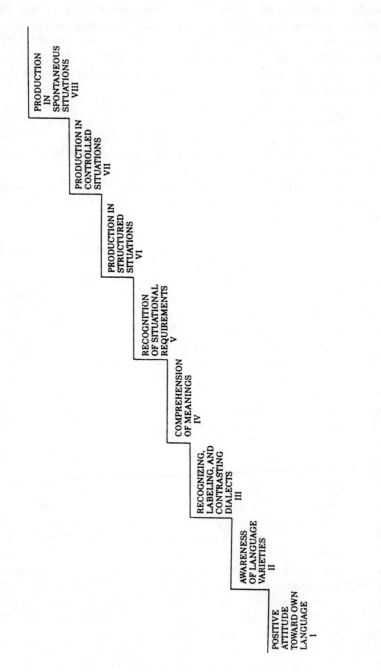

Figure 7-1. Developmental sequence of communication teaching — oral communication instruction program.

is to expose the child to a variety of forms of language. For example, stories might be read to the learner in "formal" English, poems might be written in various dialects, or records or tapes might be played that illustrate different dialects. Children might take turns retelling stories in their own dialect, with their performances tape recorded for future discussions on likenesses and differences. Young children might be taught the rules of conversation or turn-taking within their own dialect and in the second dialect through small group work, partner work, and observation. Furthermore, they could learn the effects of various nonverbal communicative behaviors by acting out their ideas.

Older SESD learners can expand their awareness of varieties of language by discussing regional and social dialects heard on television shows and by practicing the expression of their same idea for a variety of real or imagined audiences. It is important to remember, however, that at Stage II *specific* elements of likenesses and differences are not emphasized.

Step III, *recognizing, labeling,* and *contrasting dialects* may not be appropriate for very young children. If children have not yet developed to a point where they can step outside themselves and analyze the elements of what they are hearing, the process of labeling and contrasting dialects may make little sense. Older children are typically able to recognize and label specific surface structure differences between and among various dialects. However, it is unnecessary for a person to be able to label features of a dialect to acquire a competence in reproducing those features. Yet labeling can sharpen awareness and facilitate discussions among learners about the nature of language and language differences. In addition, the ability to recognize and contrast surface structure elements appears to facilitate learning of new linguistic and communicative behaviors.

Step IV in the developmental sequence, *comprehension of meanings,* can be defined narrowly as instruction that focuses on the underlying meanings (and intentions) associated with particular dialect forms. Even very young children may be aware of the fact that the same linguistic form may have different meanings if they have had an opportunity to interact with people who use different dialects. The process of communication is a kind of verbal "feeling your way" to the semantic rules of others. The greater the differences between cultural (and regional) backgrounds of listener and speaker, the greater the likelihood of significant differences in meaning. Indeed, the same utterance in two regions of a country may be interpreted as having different meanings. For example, "I need a tonic" in California is usually interpreted to mean that the speaker needs some sort of medicinal stimulant. In New England, however, the speaker would be thought to be in need of a soft drink.

Step V, *recognition of situational requirements,* involves lessons that are related to the "focus on function" already discussed. At this level, students are taught how to assess what is appropriate and inappropriate in specific communicative situations. Very young children may not be able to understand this concept fully. This inability to recognize the situational rules of communication is what makes the young child seem so straightforward, innocent, and often amusing to an adult. Older children, however, can understand what is appropriate to a given situation because they are able to anticipate the reaction of the audience in that situation. Therefore, children can be taught to use that knowledge to shape the way in which communication is used to fulfill their intentions and needs. Instruction at this stage does not require oral production by the learner, only recognition of the linguistic and communicative requirements of various situations and audiences.

Step VI, *production in structured situations,* involves lessons in which the SESD learner is given opportunities to practice the production of standard English in a situation in which the learner has some sort of assistance from the teacher—for example, a script, auditory model, or written passage (prose or poetry)—as a guide for producing standard English. Choral reading and Readers' Theatre are particularly effective teaching techniques at Step VII.

This stage of training is built around the assumption that whenever an individual learns a new linguistic behavior, imitations or productions of successive approximations of what is perceived to be the desired target are typically patterned on some sort of external model. Once approximated, the learner can then be taught how to alter and extend the original set of behaviors.

Step VII, *production in controlled situations,* involves lessons in which the student is taught to produce targeted features of the new dialect without external assistance. Role playing and story telling, for example, are excellent activities at this stage of SESD teaching. A key point to remember, however, is that the situation is controlled by the teacher and the student(s) to the extent that the communicative situation (real or imagined), audience, and intention are defined in advance, together with the communicative behaviors that are considered to be appropriate for the occasion. Step VII recognizes that a person learning a new linguistic skill can be overwhelmed by having to handle too many variables at once. By making the content and the context of the situation predictable, the teacher frees the student to concentrate more effectively on the skills being practiced.

Step VIII, the final step in the SESD developmental sequence, focuses on *production in spontaneous situation.* This step is the ultimate goal of the program. Activities are designed at this level to permit the learner to determine the linguistic and communicative requirements of a specific situation, audience, and so forth, and proceed to actual use of the required forms in a real-life experience in that situation.

IMPLEMENTING ACCPT IN THE CLASSROOM

A sample lesson from the Standard English Program Handbook (1984) of the Richmond, California, Unified School District presented in Table 7–2 demonstrates the philosophy and some of the assumptions of ACCPT, together with implementation of the eight step Developmental Sequence of Communication Teaching. The lesson is one of several that have been written and field tested by teachers in this school district, who have participated in an intensive staff development program conducted by the author of this chapter. Its focus is on specific linguistic features of standard English that typically differ in Black English vernacular.

The lesson, like all lessons in the series, represents an interactive permutation of the following factors:

1. *Feature(s) of Language:* Elements of the major components of our oral language system as defined by contemporary linguistic theory, namely:
   a. phonology
   b. semantics
   c. grammar
   d. prosody
   e. conversational postulates
   f. rhetorical and discourse styles

In the lesson presented in Table 1–2, any feature of language may be selected for instruction so long as it differs in Black English vernacular from standard English.

2. *Level(s) of Language:* One of the eight steps of the Developmental Sequence of Communication Teaching. The lesson in Table 7–2 focuses on Steps 1 through 5.

3. *Function(s):* One of the speech act categories used to classify the intentions of utterances (e.g., describing, warning, requesting). The lesson in Table 7–2 may be used for any speech act selected by the SESD teacher.

4. *Focus:* One of the three foci of the SESD Teaching Model:

Table 7-2. A Sample SESD Lesson that Uses the ACCPT Concept*

Grade Level: 4-6	Features(s) of Language: All		Level(s) of Language: 1,2,3,4,5
Function(s): All		Products: Written story	
Prerequisite(s): Awareness of one's own language		Materials needed: Books	

LEVEL OF LANGUAGE	FOCUS	DESCRIPTION OF ACTIVITY	INSTRUCTIONS	EVALUATION
I. Positive Attitude toward own language II. Awareness of language varieties III. Recognizing, Labeling Contrasting Dialects IV. Comprehension of meanings V. Recognition of situations	Recognizing the types of language *structures appropriate for a variety of people, functions, and topics*	Teacher presents versions of a story in both standard English and Black English vernacular and students *compare usage and connotations and discuss differences* (a) pattern (b) situation Teacher may rewrite a story or poem that was written in Black English vernacular	1. Teacher reads the Black English vernacular version of the story or poem and the standard English version. 2a. Teacher guides the students in discussion of how some meanings and usage may have changed from Black English vernacular to standard English. 2b. Students use partner talk to identify specific changes. 2c. Reporter from each pair shares ideas that have not already been presented with total group. 3. Teacher guides the students in discussion and understanding English is appropriate. SUGGESTED MATERIALS: • *Cornrows* by Camille Yarbrough • *Liza Lou* by Mercer Mayer • *We Be Warm Till Springtime Comes* by Lillie Chaffin	1. Have students write a short story and identify the use of Black English vernacular or standard English 2. Are students able to give examples of Black English vernacular switched to standard English? Can they explain any changes in meaning?

HOME ACTIVITY:

a. *Listen to 2 or 3 television programs (e.g., news, cartoons, and/or child's favorite program), and write or orally report on similarities and differences observed*

b. Listen to family and/or friends in various situations to note their dialect differences

*From Standard English Program Handbook (1984). Richmond, CA: Richmond Unified School District.

structure, function, and thought. The lesson in Table 7–2 is designed to focus primarily on structure and function.

There are several other characteristics that are associated with the lesson in Table 7–2. First, the lesson contains a long range "product," in this case a story to be written by members of the class. By having a product, SESD instruction is not conducted as an isolated structured activity, but rather one that is associated with a real life activity or behavior.

Second, audience and situational requirements are addressed in the lesson. This feature draws the learner's attention to the fact that the use of a particular dialect or communicative behavior is always linked to a given audience or purpose. It also gives credibility to the home dialect by emphasizing that it is quite appropriate to use it in many situations and before certain audiences.

Third, the lesson has an informal evaluation component to assess student progress or mastery. Finally, the lesson contains suggested follow-up home activities. It should be added that it is a good idea for the SESD teacher to also note how a particular activity might be integrated into various subject areas across the curriculum.

EVALUATION

Ongoing evaluation is an essential requirement of ACCPT for both the student and the teacher. At least two type of evaluation processes are recommended. The first type is a periodic evaluation of the SESD teacher's ability to implement the principles of ACCPT. This evaluation provides the teacher and the program coordinator with strengths and weaknesses of the teacher that need to be either reinforced (in the case of strengths) or improved (in the case of weaknesses). The second type of evaluation is the student's level of mastery within the context of the developmental teaching model as a function of program goals. Each of these concepts will be discussed briefly.

SESD Teacher Evauation

Teacher evaluation in ACCPT is accomplished by means of the observation checklist presented in Table 7–3. The checklist, which should be administered at least every 6 months, is built around an observation of an actual SESD lesson presented by a teacher for a real group of students.

Table 7-3. Observation Checklist for SESD Lessons*

Degree of Effectiveness

	Great 5	4	Some 3	2	Little 1	NA
1. The lesson provides an opportunity for students to give evidence of careful listening by summarizing, responding, or following directions.						
2. The lesson provides varied and frequent opportunities for students to communicate with each other.						
3. The lesson provides students with an opportunity to summarize, analyze, or evaluate oral or written materials presented by self, peers, or teacher.						
4. The lesson provides students with an opportunity to listen and respond appropriately to ideas and information presented by the teacher, by classmates, or through audiovisual materials.						
5. The lesson provides students with opportunities to use different speech acts in a variety of situations.						
6. The lesson provides students with opportunities to evaluate their own speech through a variety of informal and formal means.						
7. The lesson clearly indicates that it is attached to a short term or long term product.						
8. The lesson alerts students to the importance of situation, audience, or topic during communication.						
9. The lesson indicates that its oral communication activities will be included throughout the total curriculum.						
10. The linguistic focus of the lesson is clear.						

Observation date(s): _____

Teacher's Name: _____   Grade Level: _____

*From Standard English Program Handbook (1984). Richmond, CA: Richmond Unified School District. NA, Not Applicable.

The observation checklist requires an evaluation on a 1 to 5 rating scale of the teacher's implementation of the key elements of ACCPT in the observed lesson, if applicable. The checklist provides an assessment of teacher effectiveness for each element or across all elements. Comparisons across various points in time provide a useful index of improvement for both teacher and program coordinator.

Student Evaluations

With respect to student evaluations in the ACCPT concept, the construction of specific criterion referenced instruments is urged. These instruments are to have two major characteristics. First, the instruments should focus only on the areas of language and communication that have actually been focused on during instruction. Second, they should permit evaluation of performance at the levels of instruction that have been focused upon from the developmental Sequence of Communication Teaching presented earlier in this chapter. After all, it makes little sense — and it is unfair to the students — to assess student success on production in spontaneous situations, for example, when instruction only carried the student through production in controlled situations.

A sample criterion referenced rating scale from the aforementioned Standard English Program Handbook (1984), is presented in Table 7–4. The rating scale is based on one of the specific goals of that program for students in grades 4 through 6. The instrument should be administered on a periodic basis, probably at 6 month intervals. Like the teacher evaluation instrument, the student instrument permits both teacher and student to monitor progress in specific aspects of a goal and progress in the goal as a total unit. Based on students' response patterns, future SESD lesson planning can proceed in an orderly, goal directed manner.

Finally, SESD evaluation might make use of criterion referenced tests that focus on such items as auditory discrimination of specific standard English linguistic features that have been addressed during instruction, as well as on their production during spontaneous or nonspontaneous elicitations. Norms for such evaluations should be based on local standards. Toronto (1983) has presented an excellent summary of local norming considerations. An example of a structured elicitation approach to criterion referenced assessment of the acquisition of a specific feature of standard English is shown in Table 7–5.

Table 7–4. Sample Student Assessment of Specific Program Goal for SESD Learners: Grades 4 Through 6

DIRECTIONS: Please indicate the degree to which each student does or does not perform the following activities.

Observational Data Recording

Goal 1: Students will develop language skills that enable them to communicate effectively across cultures.

	Not At All			Very Much	NA	
1.	1	2	3	4	5	Can identify languages or dialects of different cultures within the classroom.
2.	1	2	3	4	5	Can identify and use own language or dialect.
3.	1	2	3	4	5	Can identify regional differences in speech patterns.
4.	1	2	3	4	5	Can identify differences between informal and formal language.
5.	1	2	3	4	5	Uses informal words and expressions in appropriate situations.
6.	1	2	3	4	5	Uses formal language (standard English in appropriate situations).
7.	1	2	3	4	5	Can identify differences between standard English and nonstandard English.

$$\text{Adjusted percent correct} = \frac{\text{Obtained score (total points per item)}}{\text{Maximum possible score for all applicable items (5 points per item excluding any items marked NA)}} \times 100$$

---

*From Standard English Program Handbook (1984). Richmond, CA: Richmond Unified School District.
NA, Not Applicable.

SUMMARY

This chapter has presented a discussion of background issues pertaining to the teaching of standard English as a second dialect to nonstandard English speakers and the role of the speech-language pathologist as a consultant to, or teacher in, the program. Approaches, principles, and guidelines for SESD teaching were given. Finally, a cultural and communicative approach for teaching stan-

Table 7–5.   Example of a Structured Elicitation Approach to Assess Learner's Ability to Produce a Specific Feature of Standard English*

Level___K-6___   CARD -2-   DOUBLE NEGATIVES

STANDARD ENGLISH PROFICIENCY ASSESSMENT

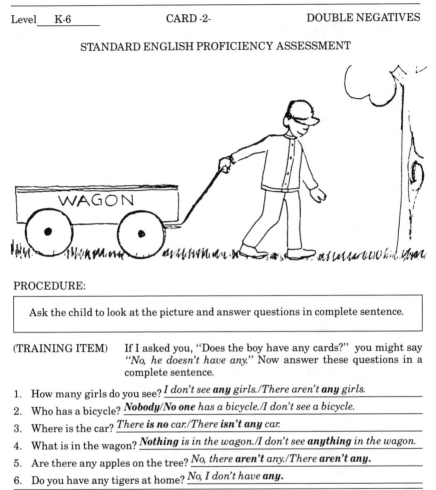

PROCEDURE:

Ask the child to look at the picture and answer questions in complete sentence.

(TRAINING ITEM)   If I asked you, "Does the boy have any cards?" you might say *"No, he doesn't have any."* Now answer these questions in a complete sentence.

1. How many girls do you see? *I don't see **any** girls./There aren't **any** girls.*

2. Who has a bicycle? *Nobody/No one has a bicycle./I don't see a bicycle.*

3. Where is the car? *There **is no** car./There **isn't any** car.*

4. What is in the wagon? *Nothing is in the wagon./I don't see **anything** in the wagon.*

5. Are there any apples on the tree? *No, there **aren't** any./There aren't **any.***

6. Do you have any tigers at home? *No, I don't have **any.***

*From Standard English Program Handbook (1984). Oakland, CA: Oakland Unified School District.

dard English while preserving the integrity and value of the learner's indigenous linguistic system has also been presented. This approach, referred to as ACCPT, has been field tested in several California cities. It is based on a developmental teaching model and contains suggestions for evaluation of both the program implementer and the student learners.

REFERENCES

Bamgbose, A. (1983). Education in indigenous languages: The West African model of language education. *Journal of Negro Education, 52,* 57–64.

Buckley, M. (1976). A guide for developing an oral language curriculum. *Language Arts, 53,* 621–627.

Craig, D. (1983). Teaching standard English to nonstandard speakers: Some methodological considerations. *Journal of Negro Education, 52,* 65–74.

Cummings, J. (1981). *Role of primary language development in promoting educational sources for language minority students.* Sacramento: California State Department of Education Compendium on Bilingual Bicultural Education.

Fasold, R. (1984). *The sociolinguistics of society.* London: Basil Blackwell.

Feigenbaum, I. (1970). The use of nonstandard English in teaching standard: Contrast and comparison. In R. Fasold and R. W. Shuy (Eds.), *Teaching standard English in the inner city.* Washington, DC: Center for Applied Linguistics.

Lau v. Nichols, 411 U. S. 563 (1974).

Martin Luther King Junior Elementary School Children et al. v. Ann Arbor School District Board, Civil Action No. 7–71861, 451 F. Supp. 1324 (1978), 463 F. Supp. 1027 (1978), and 473 F. Supp. 1371 (1979) (Detroit, Michigan, July 12, 1979).

Saville-Troike, M. (1982). *The ethnography of communication.* Baltimore: University Park Press.

Standard English Program Handbook (1984). Richmond, CA: Richmond Unified School District.

Standards for Effective Oral Communications Programs (n.d.). Unpublished document by American Speech and Hearing Association (Rockville, MD) and Speech Communication Association (Annandale, VA).

Taylor, O. L., Stroud, R. V., Hurst, C. G., Moore, E. J., and Williams, R. (1969). Philosophies and goals of the ASHA Black Caucus: A special report. *ASHA, II,* 221–225.

Toronto, A. S. (1983). Developing locally normed assessment instruments. In D. R. Omark and J. G. Erickson (Eds.), *The bilingual exceptional child.* San Diego: College-Hill Press.

Postscript:

Where Do We Go from Here?

In this book, we have explored several issues pertaining to culturally and linguistically valid assessment and treatment procedures for communication disorders in several groups in the United States. We have also presented a cultural and communication based approach for teaching standard English as a second dialect. This approach can be used by classroom teachers or by speech pathologists working in a teaching or consultative capacity.

Now the question is "Where do we go from here?" First, we must obviously conduct more research on clinical issues in communication disorders as they pertain to the various cultural and linguistic groups that reside in the United States, or even the world. This research should pay special attention to groups given little attention in this book (e.g., Asian Americans). Second, increased research activity is also needed on second language and dialect teaching and acquisition.

If the reader has not already done so, he or she should read the companion volume, *Nature of Communication Disorders in Culturally and Linguistically Diverse Populations* for better understanding of theoretical issues and data on this subject. Based on the discussions in these two books, it is obvious that cultural and linguistic diversity issues have acquired a legitimate place within the field of communication disorders and are fruitful subjects for research and clinical practice.

Appendix A

Position of the American Speech-Language-Hearing Association on Social Dialects*

The English language is comprised of many linguistic varieties, such as Black English,* standard English, Appalachian English, southern English, New York dialect, and Spanish influenced English. The features of social dialects are systematic and highly regular and cross all linguistic

parameters, i.e., phonology, morphology, syntax, semantics, lexicon, pragmatics, suprasegmental features, and kinesics. Although each dialect of English has distinguishing characteristics, the majority of linguistic features of the English language are common to each of the varieties of English. The existence of these varieties is the result of historical and social factors. For example, due to historical factors, the majority of Black English speakers are Black. However, due to social factors, not all Black individuals are Black English speakers.

The issue of social dialects for the field of speech-language pathology is extremely complex as indicated by the continuous controversy across the nation over the past two decades. There has been confusion among professionals regarding the role of the speech-language pathologist with reference to speakers of social dialects. There has been no consistent philosophy regarding the approach of service delivery to speakers of social dialects. As a result, some speech-language pathologists have denied clinical services to speakers of social dialects who have requested services. Other speech-language pathologists have treated social dialects as though they were communicative disorders.

It is the position of the American Speech-Language-Hearing Association (ASHA) that no dialectal variety of English is a disorder or a pathological form of speech or language. Each social dialect is adequate as a functional and effective variety of English. Each serves a communication function as well as a social solidarity function. It maintains the communication network and the social construct of the community of speakers who use it. Furthermore, each is a symbolic representation of the historical, social, and cultural background of the speakers. For example, there is strong evi-

---

*Some Black professionals prefer to use the terms Ebonics instead of the more popularly used term Black English. Derived from the words *ebony* and *phonics,* the term Ebonics is intended to avoid the focus on race and emphasize the ethnolinguistic origin and evolution of this variety of the English language.

dence that many of the features of Black English represent linguistic Africanisms.

However, society has adopted the linguistic idealization model that standard English is the linguistic archetype. Standard English is the linguistic variety used by government, the mass media, business, education, science, and the arts. Therefore, there may be nonstandard English speakers who find it advantageous to have access to the use of standard English.

The traditional role of the speech-language pathologist has been to provide clinical services to the communicatively handicapped. It is indeed possible for dialect speakers to have linguistic disorders within the dialect. An essential step toward making accurate assessments of communicative disorders is to distinguish between those aspects of linguistic variation that represent the diversity of the English language from those that represent speech, language, and hearing disorders. The speech-language pathologist must have certain competencies to distinguish between dialectal differences and communicative disorders. These competencies include knowledge of the particular dialect as a rule-governed linguistic system, knowledge of the phonological and grammatical features of the dialect, and knowledge of nondiscriminatory testing procedures. Once the difference-disorder distinctions have been made, it is the role of the speech-language pathologist to treat only those features or characteristics that are true errors and not attributable to the dialect.

Aside from the traditionally recognized role, the speech-language pathologist may also be available to provide *elective* clinical services to nonstandard English speakers who do not present a disorder. The role of the speech-language pathologist for these individuals is to provide the desired competency in standard English without jeopardizing the integrity of the individual's first dialect. The approach must be functional and based on context-specific appropriateness of the given dialect.

Provision of elective services to nonstandard English speakers requires sensitivity and competency in at least three areas: linguistic features of the dialect, linguistic contrastive analysis procedures, and the effects of attitudes toward dialects. It is prerequisite for the speech-language pathologist to have a thorough understanding and appreciation for the community and culture of the nonstandard English speaker. Further, it is a requirement that the speech-language pathologist have thorough knowledge of the linguistic rules of the particular dialect.

It remains the priority of the speech-language pathologist to continue to serve the truly communicatively handicapped. However, for nonstandard English speakers who seek elective clinical services, the speech-language pathologist may also serve in a consultative role to assist educators in utilizing the features of the nonstandard dialect to facilitate the learning of reading and writing in standard English. Just as competencies are assumed and necessary in the treatment of communicative disorders, competencies are also necessary in the provision of elective clinical services to nonstandard English speakers.

From ASHA, September 1983, pp. 23–25.

Appendix B

Standards for Effective Oral Communication Programs

prepared by

American Speech-Language-Hearing Association and Speech Communication Association

Adequate oral communication frequently determines an individual's educational, social, and vocational success. Yet, American education has typically neglected formal instruction in the basic skills of speaking and listening. It is important that state and local education agencies implement the most effective oral communication programs possible.

The following standards for oral communication were developed by representatives of the Speech Communication Association and the American Speech-Language-Hearing Association.

If effective oral communication programs are going to be developed, all components of the recommended standards must be considered. Implementation of these standards will facilitate development of adequate and appropriate oral communication necessary for educational, social, and vocational success.

DEFINITION

Oral Communication: The process of interacting through heard and spoken messages in a variety of situations.

Effective oral communication is a learned behavior, involving the following processes:

1. Speaking in a variety of educational and social situations: Speaking involves, but is not limited to, arranging and producing messages through the use of voice, articulation, vocabulary, syntax, and nonverbal cues (e.g., gesture, facial expression, vocal cues) appropriate to the speaker and listeners.
2. Listening in a variety of educational and social situations: Listening involves, but is not limited to, hearing, perceiving, discriminating, inter-

preting, synthesizing, evaluating, organizing, and remembering information from verbal and nonverbal messages.

BASIC ASSUMPTIONS

1. Oral communication behaviors of students can be improved through direct instruction.
2. Oral communication instruction emphasizes the interactive nature of speaking and listening.
3. Oral communication instruction addresses the everyday communication needs of students and includes emphasis on the classroom as a practical communication environment.
4. There is a wide range of communication competence among speakers of the same language.
5. Communication competence is not dependent upon use of a particular form of language.
6. A primary goal of oral communication instruction is to increase the students' repertoire and use of effective speaking and listening behaviors.
7. Oral communication programs provide instruction based on a coordinated developmental continuum of skills, preschool through adult.
8. Oral communication skills can be enhanced by using parents, supportive personnel, and appropriate instructional technology.

AN EFFECTIVE COMMUNICATION PROGRAM HAS THE FOLLOWING CHARACTERISTICS

Teaching, Learning

1. The oral communication program is based on current theory and research in speech and language development, psycholinguistics, rhetorical and communication theory, communication disorders, speech science, and related fields of study.
2. Oral communication instruction is a clearly identifiable part of the curriculum.
3. Oral communication instruction is systematically related to reading and writing instruction and to instruction in the various content areas.
4. The relevant academic, personal, and social experiences of students provide core subject matter for the oral communication program.
5. Oral communication instruction provides a wide range of speaking and listening experience, in order to develop effective communication skills appropriate to:
   a. a range of situations; e.g., informal to formal, interpersonal to mass communication.
   b. a range of purposes; e.g., informing, learning, persuading, evaluating messages, facilitating social interaction, sharing feelings, imaginative and creative expression.
   c. a range of audiences; e.g., classmates, teachers, peers, employers, family, community.

    d. a range of communication forms; e.g., conversation, group discussion, interview, drama, debate, public speaking, oral interpretation.

    e. a range of speaking styles; impromptu, extemporaneous, and reading from manuscript.

6. The oral communication program provides class time for systematic instruction in oral communication skills, e.g., critical listening, selecting, arranging and presenting messages, giving and receiving constructive feedback, non-verbal communication, etc.

7. The oral communication program includes development of adequate and appropriate language, articulation, voice, fluency, and listening skills necessary for success in educational, career, and social situations through regular classroom instruction, cocurricular activities, and speech-language pathology and audiology services.

8. Oral communication program instruction encourages and provides appropriate opportunities for the reticent student (e.g., one who is excessively fearful in speaking situations) to participate more effectively in oral communication.

SUPPORT

1. Oral communication instruction is provided by individuals adequately trained in oral communication or communication disorders, as evidenced by appropriate certification.

2. Individuals responsible for oral communication instruction receive continuing education on theories, research, and instruction relevant to communication.

3. Individuals responsible for oral communication instruction participate actively in conventions, meetings, publications, and other activities of communication professionals.

4. The oral communication program includes a system for training classroom teachers to identify and refer students who do not have adequate listening and speaking skills, or are reticent, to those qualified individuals who can best meet the needs of the student through further assessment or instruction, or both.

5. Teachers in all curriculum areas receive information on appropriate methods for: (a) using oral communication to facilitate instruction, and (b) using the subject matter to improve students' oral communication skills.

6. Parent and community groups are informed about and provided with appropriate materials for effective involvement in the oral communication program.

7. The oral communication program is facilitated by availability and use of appropriate instructional materials, equipment, and facilities.

ASSESSMENT AND EVALUATION

1. The oral communication program is based on a schoolwide assessment of the speaking and listening needs of students.

2. Speaking and listening needs of students will be determined by qualified personnel utilizing appropriate evaluation tools for the skills to be assessed and educational levels of students being assessed.
3. Evaluation of student progress in oral communication is based upon a variety of data, including observations, self-evaluations, listeners' responses to messages, and formal tests.
4. Evaluation of students' oral communication encourages, rather than discourages, students' desires to communicate by emphasizing those behaviors that students can improve, thus enhancing their ability to do so.
5. Evaluation of the total communication program is based on achievement of acceptable levels of oral communication skill determined by continuous monitoring of student progress in speaking and listening, use of standardized and criterion-referenced tests, audience-based rating scales, and other appropriate instruments.

Appendix C

Clinical Management of Communicatively Handicapped Minority Language Populations

Prepared by

American Speech-Language-Hearing Association

STATEMENT OF NEED

The special needs of minority language populations (native speakers of languages other than English) were the source of national controversy even before the Bilingual Education Act was enacted nearly two decades ago. Professionals in bilingual education, regular education, special education, linguistics, sociology, second language instruction, psychology, learning disabilities, as well as speech-language pathology and audiology, have debated innumerable issues, approaches, theories, and philosophical positions regarding minority language populations. As a result of this wide-spread controversy, there has been considerable confusion among these various professionals concerning this population.

According to the 1980 Census, 34.6 million or 15 percent of the U.S. population is composed of native speakers of various minority languages. It is estimated by ASHA that approximately 3.5 million of these speakers have speech, language, or hearing disorders that are unrelated to the use of a minority language. Researchers and clinicians are only beginning to amass a knowledge base on the characteristics of normal language development in various minority languages, bilingual language learning, second language acquisition, dominance testing, bilingual assessment and remediation of communicative disorders, and the applications of emerging computer technology for use with minority language groups. Therefore, it would be premature to propose in this paper optimum strategies for identification, assessment, and intervention.

However, it *is* firmly established that most ASHA members are aware of their limitations in language proficiency and in their knowledge of diverse cultures which restrict their competence to serve minority language populations. According to the 1982 ASHA Self Study Survey, 77 percent of the certified speech-language pathologists indicated a need for more knowledge and skill to serve bilingual-bicultural populations. Given that the minority language population is ever increasing, there is an immediate need for professionals to either upgrade their own levels of competence or to employ alternative strategies to address the needs of the communicatively handicapped among the various minority language populations. Thus, it is the purpose of this paper to recommend competencies for assessment and remediation of communicative disorders of minority language speakers and to describe alternative strategies that can be utilized when those competencies are not met.

It is obvious that assessment and remediation of some disorders of communication are not hampered by the client's use of a minority language. For example, assessment of pure tone hearing thresholds, auditory brainstem response, acoustic reflexes, and other similar services may not necessitate much communicative exchange between the examiner and the client. Likewise, assessment of the physical support for speech, assessment of anomalies affecting speech such as cleft lip and palate, palatal insufficiency, oral malocclusion, etc., also may be conducted without proficiency in the minority language. These examples are by no means exhaustive, but are provided to emphasize that there are clinical services that can be provided appropriately by a monolingual English professional to a minority language speaker. However, because the effectiveness of the professional is dependent on interpersonal skill in addition to technical skill the overall professional client relationship is affected when communication is limited.

For many other aspects of speech, language, and hearing, assessment and remediation are much more complicated by the client's use of a minority language. For example, the phonemic, allophonic, syntactic, morphological, semantic, lexical, and pragmatic characteristics of a minority language cannot be adequately assessed or remediated without knowledge of that language. Further, auditory discrimination and speech reception thresholds may be difficult to assess without the ability to test in the minority language.

Voice qualities, such as harshness, breathiness, loudness, pitch, and the production of clicks and glottal stops, vary across languages. These factors may make it difficult to rule out vocal pathology when the examiner is unfamiliar with the vocal characteristics common to a given language.

Hesitations, false starts, filled and silent pauses, and other dysfluent behavior may be exhibited by a bilingual speaker due to lack of familiarity with English. Thus, differential diagnosis of true stuttering from normal dysfluency may be difficult if the examiner is unfamiliar with the client's use of the minority language.

Identification of prosodic or suprasegmental problems is extremely difficult if the examiner is not familiar with the prosodic characteristics of the minority language. Even when the examiner is familiar with the given language, dialect differences *within* that language may be a confounding variable in assessment.

There are also cultural variables that may influence how speech-language pathology and audiology services are accepted by minority language populations. Differences between minority cultures and the general population in traditions, customs, values, beliefs, and practices may affect service delivery. Thus, speech-language pathologists and audiologists must provide services with consideration of such cultural variables, in addition to consideration of language differences.

Thus, it is apparent that the assessment and remediation of many aspects of speech, language, and hearing of minority language speakers require specific background and skills. This is not only logical and sound clinical practice, but it is the consensus set forth by federal mandates such as The Education for All Handicapped Children Act of 1975 (PL 94-142) and The Bilingual Education Act of 1976 (PL 95-561: Title VII of the Elementary and Secondary Education Act of 1965); legal decisions such as Dianna v. Board of Education (1973), Lau v. Nichols (1974), Larry P. v. Riles (1977) and the Martin Luther King Junior Elementary School Children v. Ann Arbor School District Board (1979); and the policies and practices of many professional agencies and organizations such as the National Association for Bilingual Education, the National Center for Bilingual Research, the Center for Applied Linguistics, and the National Hispanic Psychological Association.

Even state regulations are being developed to acknowledge the need for specific competencies to serve minority language populations. In California, for example, school districts are being encouraged by the State Education Agency to require resource specialists, speech-language pathologists and school psychologists to pass a state administered oral and written examination on Hispanic culture, Spanish language, and assessment methodology before they conduct assessments for Spanish-speaking children with limited English proficiency. Other states and U.S. territories with education legislation which addresses the special needs of minority language populations include Alaska, American Samoa, Arizona, Colorado,

Connecticut, Indiana, Iowa, Kansas, Maine, Massachusetts, Michigan, Minnesota, New Hampshire, New Jersey, New Mexico, Oregon, Puerto Rico, South Dakota, Tennessee, Texas, Territory of the Pacific Islands, Utah, Vermont, Washington, Wisconsin, and Wyoming (American Speech-Language-Hearing Association, 1982).

CONTINUUM OF LANGUAGE PROFICIENCY

There are scores of different minority languages spoken in the United States. But within each group of minority language speakers there is also a continuum of proficiency in English. In provision of services to minority language speakers with communicative disorders, the continuum is particularly relevant. The continuum includes speakers who are:
- Bilingual English Proficient,
- Limited English Proficient,
- Limited in both English and the Minority language.

Depending on the client's English language proficiency on the continuum, recommended competencies for the professional are:

Competencies

Bilingual English Proficient

There are bilingual individuals who are fluent in English. Those who have greater control of English than the minority language individuals can be regarded as bilingual English proficient.

For individuals who are bilingual English proficient and evidence a communicative disorder in English, it is *not* essential that the speech-language pathologist or audiologist be proficient in the minority language to provide assessment and remediation in *English*. However, the speech-language pathologist must attain certain competencies to distinguish between dialectal differences (due to interaction from the minority language) and communicative disorders. These competencies include understanding the minority language as a rule-governed system, knowledge of the correct phonological, grammatical, semantic, and pragmatic features of the minority language, and knowledge of nondiscriminatory procedures (refer to "Social Dialects: A Position Paper," *ASHA*, September 1983).

Limited English Proficient

Some bilingual individuals and monolingual individuals are proficient in their native language but not in English. Assessment and intervention of speech and language disorders of limited English proficient speakers should be conducted in the client's primary language. This is consistent with federal mandates (PL 94-142 and Title VII of PL 95-561), legal decisions (such as *Dianna v. Board of Education, Lau v. Nichols,* and *Larry P. v. Riles*), and the education regulations of many states.

To provide assessment and remediation services *in the minority language,* it is recommended that the speech-language pathologist or audiologist possess the following competencies:

Language Proficiency: Native or near native fluency in both the minority language and the English language.

Normative Processes. Ability to describe the process of normal speech and language acquisition for both bilingual and monolingual individuals; and how those processes are manifested in oral and written language.

Assessment: Ability to administer and interpret formal and informal assessment procedures to distinguish between communication difference and communication disorders.

Intervention: Ability to apply intervention strategies for treatment of communicative disorders in the minority language.

Cultural Sensitivity: Ability to recognize cultural factors which affect the delivery of speech-language pathology and audiology services to minority language speaking community.

Limited in Both Languages

There are bilingual individuals who are truly communicatively handicapped, possessing limited communicative competence in both languages. For such individuals, speech and language should be assessed in both languages to determine language dominance. Thus, the same competencies listed for limited English proficient speakers are recommended for assessment for this group of speakers. The most appropriate language for intervention would be determined from the assessment.

If the most appropriate language for intervention is the minority language, then the competencies recommended for serving limited

English proficient speakers should be met to provide therapy. If the most appropriate language for intervention is English, proficiency in the minority language may not be necessary to provide therapy.

It is important to note that the determination of bilingual dominance in communicatively handicapped individuals may be particularly difficult. It is stressed that both objectives and subjective measures should be utilized to determine if the client's dominant language is either English or the minority language.

Alternative Strategies for Use of Professional Personnel

It is recognized that not all speech-language pathologists and audiologists possess the recommended competencies to serve limited English proficient speakers. Following are some strategies for procuring speech-language pathologists who do meet the aforementioned competencies when there are none on staff.

1. **Establish Contacts.** Bilingual speech-language pathologists or audiologists can be hired by school districts and other clinical programs as consultants to evaluate and remediate minority language speakers on an as needed basis.
2. **Establish Cooperative.** A clinical cooperative can be developed to allow a group of school districts or clinical programs to hire an itinerant bilingual speech-language pathologist or audiologist whose primary responsibility is to serve a specific minority language population.
3. **Establish Networks.** Strong ties could be established between professional work settings and university programs that have bilingual speech-language pathology or audiology programs so that there can be an interchange of existing resources. Once such a liaison is established, it can facilitate recruitment of speech-language pathologists or audiologists who are competent to serve minority language populations after they graduate.
4. **Establish CFY and Graduate Practicum Sites.** Graduate students or recent graduates from bilingual communicative disorders programs, under the direct supervision of a bilingual speech-language pathologist or audiologist, could be used to assist personnel in schools and other clinical facilities in assessment and intervention of limited English-proficient individuals.
5. **Establish Interdisciplinary Teams.** A team approach can be implemented which includes the monolingual speech-language pathologist or audiologist and a bilingual professional equal (e.g., psychologist, special education teacher, etc.) who is knowl-

edgeable of non-biased assessment procedures and language development of the particular minority language.

An agency contracting the services of a speech-language pathologist or audiologist to serve limited English-proficient speakers may not be in a position to evaluate the professional's competencies. Therefore, when employing the preceding alternative strategies, efforts should be made to assure that the speech-language pathologist or audiologist is competent to serve a given minority language population.

Use of Interpreters or Translators

Interpreters or translators could be used with minority language speakers when the following circumstances exist: (a) when the certified speech-language pathologist or audiologist on the staff does not meet the recommended competencies to provide services to limited-English proficient speakers; (b) when an individual who needs services speaks a language which is uncommon for that local area; and (c) when there are no trained professionals readily available with proficiency in that language that would permit the use of one of the previously described alternative strategies. Individuals who could serve as interpreters or translators can include (1) professional interpreters from language banks or professional interpreting services, (2) bilingual professional staff from a health or education discipline other than communicative disorders, or (3) a family member or friend of the client.

If the use of interpreters or translators is the only alternative, the speech-language pathologist or audiologist should:

1. Provide extensive training to the assistant on the purposes, procedures and goals of the tests and therapy methods. The assistant also should be taught to avoid the use of gestures, vocal intonation, and other cues that could inadvertently alert the individual to the correct response during test administration.
2. Pre-plan for an individual's services to insure the assistant's understanding of specific clinical procedures to be used.
3. Use the same assistant(s) with a given minority language client rather than using assistants on a random basis.
4. Use patient observation or other non-linguistic measures as supplements to the translated measures, such as (1) child's interaction with parents, (2) child's interaction with peers, (3) pragmatic analysis.

It is recommended that the speech-language pathologist and audiologist state in their written evaluations that a translator was used and the validity of the results may be affected.

FUTURE DIRECTIONS

It is stressed that the competencies and alternative strategies delineated herein are interim in an effort to address the crisis that presently exists in the delivery of services to minority language populations. Therefore, these competencies and alternative strategies may be subject to revision or expansion as our professional knowledge base continues to increase. In addition to promoting the continued advancement of knowledge, it should be the ultimate goal of the profession to increase the percentage of speech-language pathologists and audiologists who are competent to serve minority language populations. This can be accomplished by 1) stimulating bilingual student recruitment efforts, 2) promoting relevant continuing education activities and, 3) promoting the topic of minority language populations within professional education.

The establishment of competencies in the area of service delivery to minority language populations is not intended to impose prohibitions or a hands-off philosophy for those who do not meet those competencies. But it is the professional responsibility of the speech-language pathologist and audiologist to judge their own minority language proficiency, clinical knowledge base, and cultural sensitivity in terms of the competencies delineated in this paper. Where there are deficiencies that can be reversed, it is incumbent on professionals to upgrade their level of competence through professional and continuing education programs, independent study of the growing literature on minority language populations, and ongoing involvement within the community of minority language speakers. Otherwise alternative strategies should be implemented to serve minority language speakers.

Because the competencies and alternative strategies discussed in this paper are interim, multicultural research and continued development of techniques and materials for assessment and intervention need to be priorities of professionals who provide service to these populations. Professionals also should stimulate further development and implementation of creative alternatives in order to provide appropriate and effective speech-language pathology and audiology services to minority language speakers.

REFERENCES

American Speech-Language-Hearing Association (1982). *Urban and ethnic perspectives,* October, 9–10.

Dianna v. State Board of Education, C.A. 70 RFT (N.D. Cal., Feb. 3, 1970).

Larry P. v. Riles, Civil Action No. 0-71-2270, 343 F. Supp. 1306 (N.D. Cal., 1972).

Lau v. Nichols, 411 U.S. 563 (1974).

Martin Luther King Junior Elementary School Children, et al. v. Ann Arbor School District Board, Civil Action No. 7-71861, 451 F. Supp. 1324 (1978), 463 F. Supp. 1027 (1978) and 473 F. Supp. 1371 (1979) (Detroit, Michigan, July 12, 1979).

Social dialects: A position paper (1983). *ASHA, 25(9),* 23–24.

Public Law 94-142, The Education of All Handicapped Children Act (Nov. 29, 1975).

Public Law 95-561, The Bilingual Education Act (Title VII of the Elementary and Secondary Education Act of 1965).

Appendix D

A Sample Lesson For Teaching Standard English as a Second Dialect Which Utilizes Bilingual Education Approach*

INSTRUCTIONAL FOCUS: Possessives (Morpheme -s with nouns)

OBJECTIVE: Given structured drill and practice contrasting *the use of possessive nouns,* the students will be able to differentiate between standard and nonstandard usage and to formulate sentences using the standard form in response to statements or questions.

LEVEL: Teacher Judgment

MATERIAL: A. Pair of multiple response cards labeled same and different for each student.

               B. Pair of multiple response cards labeled standard and nonstandard.

PROCEDURES:

1. To assess the students' abilities in auditory discrimination, the teacher will lead the students in the following drill. Students will respond by displaying a *same* or *different* response card.

DISCRIMINATION DRILL:

Teacher Stimulus	*Student Response*
• This is Joe car. This is Joe's car.	• different
• That is Steve's house. That is Steve's house.	• same
• This is Monika's jump rope. This is Monika jump rope.	• different

---

*From Standard English Program, Oakland (CA) Unified School District (1984).

198 Communication Disorders in Culturally Diverse Populations

- Where is Jim's skateboard?
  Where is Jim's skateboard?
- same

- Is that Doug's football?
  Is that Doug's football?
- same

- There is Pam's school.
  There is Pam school.
- different

2. The teacher will explain and model the standard form and have students repeat several examples giving additional help where needed.

3. The teacher will lead the students in the following drill. Students will respond by displaying standard or nonstandard response cards.

IDENTIFICATION DRILL:

- Mary brother is little.   Nonstandard
- Bill store is closed.   Nonstandard
- Tom's truck is red.   Standard
- Ted frog jumps high.   Nonstandard
- Jerome's cat is gray.   Standard
- Terry bicycle goes fast.   Nonstandard
- Jackie's coat is blue.   Standard
- Kevin lunch box is black.   Nonstandard

4. To check for understanding the teacher will call on individual students to respond to questions and statements similar to those in the following drill. Students will respond in complete sentences using the standard form. Students should be instructed to listen for only one nonstandard feature and to respond in complete sentences. Contractions are acceptable.

TRANSLATION DRILL:

Teacher Stimulus	*Student Response*
• Jesse truck is red.	• Jesse's truck is red.
• Monica school is large.	• Monica's school is large
• Larry jacket is black and brown.	• Larry's jacket is black and brown.
• Brian mother is ill.	• Brian's mother is ill

5. In the following drill the students will generate their own sentences in response to the teacher stimulus. The student responses listed here are but examples.

Students should be instructed to respond in complete sentences, although sometimes in everyday speech we do not. Contractions are acceptable.

RESPONSE DRILLS:

Teacher Stimulus	*Student Response*
• Is that Jessie house?	• Yes, that is Jessie's house.
• Is that John mother?	• No, that is not John's mother.
• Are those Monica skates?	• Yes, those are Monica's skates.
• That is Tobby milk.	• No, that is not Tobby's milk.
• Where are Jerry shoes?	• Here are Jerry's shoes.
• Where is Cassandra coat?	• Cassandra's coat is hanging on the hook.

EXPANSION ACTIVITY (General):

A. Guide students in reading the narrative from the life of Charles Richard Drew (see attached). Discuss content.

B. Direct attention to the italicized phrases. Elicit oral translation phrases. Elicit oral translations of these phrases into possessive form. Example:

The dream of Charles Drew would be *Charles Drew's dream*

C. After working through the entire story orally with students, provide independent practice by having them rewrite the story, translating all the phrases to the standard possessive form. Papers may be exchanged and read for peer evaluation.

EXPANSION: (Upper Grades) — Science/Health/Careers/Black History:

A. Have students research and report on the career of Daniel Hale Williams. How was his career similar to that of Charles Drew?

B. Study the circulatory system for a better understanding of the contributions of both these men to the medical profession.

C. List various medical professions and do research to find out more about them. This may be done through student interviews or by inviting persons from medical professions to speak to the class.

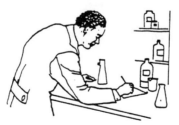

CHARLES RICHARD DREW

The dream of Charles Drew was to become a doctor. He attended Amherst College, but *the courses at this school* did not prepare him to become a doctor. Charles taught for two years to earn money for medical school.

As a doctor, *the interests of this young man* were in blood and blood transfusions. A transfusion is the passing of blood *from the veins of one person to the veins of another.* Dr. Drew discovered a way to change plasma, *the liquid part of the* blood, to powder. This way it could be stored and sent long distances. During World War II, the *wounds of injured soldiers* were treated with this powder. It saved *the lives of many men.* Dr. Drew also learned that *the skin of a person* had nothing to do with blood. All people are alike under the skin.

Because of *the interests of Dr. Drew* in blood, he got the idea of starting a blood bank. Here people could borrow blood when needed. *This idea, spun by Dr. Charles Drew,* caused him to be known as "Father of the Blood Bank."

Author Index

Subject Index

(t) following page number indicates a table